Lecture Notes in Computer Science   8040

Commenced Publication in 1973
Founding and Former Series Editors:
Gerhard Goos, Juris Hartmanis, and Jan van Leeuwen

Daniel Zeng   Christopher C. Yang
Vincent S. Tseng   Chunxiao Xing
Hsinchun Chen   Fei-Yue Wang
Xiaolong Zheng (Eds.)

Smart Health

International Conference, ICSH 2013
Beijing, China, August 3-4, 2013
Proceedings

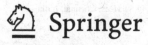 Springer

Volume Editors

Daniel Zeng
The University of Arizona, Tucson, AZ, USA
and Chinese Academy of Sciences, Beijing, China
E-mail: zeng@email.arizona.edu

Christopher C. Yang
Drexel University, Philadelphia, PA, USA
E-mail: chris.yang@drexel.edu

Vincent S. Tseng
Taiwan National Cheng Kung University, Tainan, Taiwan
E-mail: tsengsm@mail.ncku.edu.tw

Chunxiao Xing
Tsinghua University, Beijing, China
E-mail: xingcx@tsinghua.edu.cn

Hsinchun Chen
The University of Arizona, Tucson, AZ, USA
E-mail: hchen@eller.arizona.edu

Fei-Yue Wang
Chinese Academy of Sciences, Beijing, China
E-mail: feiyue.wang@ia.ac.cn

Xiaolong Zheng
Chinese Academy of Sciences, Beijing, China
E-mail: xiaolong.zheng@ia.ac.cn

ISSN 0302-9743   e-ISSN 1611-3349
ISBN 978-3-642-39843-8   e-ISBN 978-3-642-39844-5
DOI 10.1007/978-3-642-39844-5
Springer Heidelberg Dordrecht London New York

Library of Congress Control Number: Applied for

CR Subject Classification (1998): H.2, H.3.1-6, H.4, H.5

LNCS Sublibrary: SL 3 – Information Systems and Application, incl. Internet/Web and HCI

Typesetting: Camera-ready by author, data conversion by Scientific Publishing Services, Chennai, India
Printed on acid-free paper
Springer is part of Springer Science+Business Media (www.springer.com)

Preface

Significant effort has been made to advance informatics for healthcare and health-care applications. Emphasis is increasingly being placed on transforming reactive care to proactive and preventive care, clinic-centric to patient-centered practice, training-based interventions to globally aggregated evidence, and episodic response to continuous well-being monitoring and maintenance.

The 2013 International Conference for Smart Health (ICSH) was organized to develop a platform for authors to discuss fundamental principles, algorithms or applications of intelligent data acquisition, processing and analysis of health-care data. We are pleased that many high-quality papers were submitted, including technical contributions, accompanied by evaluation with real-world data or application contexts. The work presented at the conference encompassed a healthy mix of computer science, medical informatics, and information systems approaches.

ICSH 2013 was held in Beijing, China. The 1.5-day event, including presentations of 15 papers, was co-located with the 23rd International Joint Conference on Artificial Intelligence (IJCAI 2013).

The organizers of ICSH 2013 would like to thank the conference sponsors for their support and sponsorship, including the Chinese Academy of Sciences, Chinese Military Academy of Health Sciences, Beijing Centers for Disease Control and Prevention (CDC), and University of Arizona. We also greatly appreciate the following technical co-sponsors: the Institute of Electrical and Electronics Engineers (IEEE) Computational Intelligence Society, IEEE Systems, Man, and Cybernetics Society, Institute for Operations Research and the Management Sciences (INFORMS) Artificial Intelligence College, ACM Beijing Chapter, International Federation of Automatic Control (IFAC) Economic and Business Systems Technical Committee, and Chinese Association of Automation. We further wish to express our sincere gratitude to all the workshop Program Committee members, who provided valuable and constructive review comments.

July 2013

Daniel Zeng
Christopher C. Yang
Vincent S. Tseng
Chunxiao Xing
Hsinchun Chen
Fei-Yue Wang
Xiaolong Zheng

Organizing Committee

Conference Co-chairs

Hsinchun Chen   University of Arizona, USA
Fei-Yue Wang   Chinese Academy of Sciences, China

Program Co-chairs

Daniel Zeng   University of Arizona and Chinese Academy
     of Sciences, USA/China
Christopher C. Yang   Drexel University, USA
Vincent S. Tseng   National Cheng Kung University, Taiwan
Chunxiao Xing   Tsinghua University, China

Local Arrangements Committee Co-chairs

Hongbin Song   Chinese Military Academy of Health Sciences,
     China
Quanyi Wang   Beijing Centers for Diseases Control and
     Prevention, China

Tutorial Co-chairs

John Brownstein   Harvard Medical School, USA
Daniel Neill   Carnegie Mellon University, USA

Publication Co-chairs

Wendy Chapman   University of California, San Diego, USA
Scott Leischow   Mayo Clinic, USA
Hsin-Min Lu   National Taiwan University, Taiwan
Xiaolong Zheng   Chinese Academy of Sciences, China

Poster Chair

Howard Burkom   Johns Hopkins University, USA

Finance Co-chairs

Xue-Wen Chen   Wayne State University, USA
Zhidong Cao   Chinese Academy of Sciences, China

Publicity Co-chairs

Jim Hendler	Rensselaer Polytechnic Institute, USA
Leslie Lenert	University of Utah, USA
Kwok Tsui	City University of Hong Kong, SAR China

Program Committee

Yigal Arens	University of Southern California, USA
Ian Brooks	University of Illinois at Urbana-Champaign, USA
David Buckeridge	McGill University, Canada
Nitesh V. Chawla	University of Notre Dame, USA
Guanling Chen	University of Massachusetts Lowell, USA
Kup-Sze Choi	The Hong Kong Polytechnic University, SAR China
Kainan Cui	Chinese Academy of Sciences, China
Amar Das	Dartmouth College, USA
Ron Fricker	Naval Postgraduate School, USA
Hassan Ghasemzadeh	University of California, Los Angeles, USA
Natalia Grabar	STL CNRS Université Lille 3, France
Takahiro Hara	Osaka University, Japan
Saike He	Chinese Academy of Sciences, China
Xiaohua Hu	Drexel University, USA
Kun Huang	The Ohio State University, USA
Roozbeh Jafari	University of Texas at Dallas, USA
Ernesto Jimenez-Ruiz	University of Oxford, UK
Victor Jin	The Ohio State University, USA
Hung-Yu Kao	National Cheng Kung University, Taiwan
Kenneth Komatsu	Arizona Department of Health Services, USA
Erhun Kundakcioglu	University of Houston, USA
Feipei Lai	National Taiwan University, Taiwan
Gondy Leroy	Claremont Graduate University, USA
Jiao Li	Chinese Academy of Medical Sciences, China
Xiaoli Li	Institute for Infocomm Research, Singapore
Chuan Luo	Chinese Academy of Sciences, China
Mohammad Mahoor	University of Denver, USA
Jin-Cheon Na	Nanyang Technological University, Singapore
Radhakrishnan Nagarajan	University of Kentucky, USA
Balakrishnan Prabhakaran	University of Texas at Dallas, USA
Xiaoming Sheng	University of Utah, USA
Min Song	New Jersey Institute of Technology, USA
Xing Tan	University of Ottawa, Canada
Chunqiang Tang	IBM Research
Cui Tao	Mayo Clinic, USA

Table of Contents

Smart Health Applications

Portrayal of Electronic Cigarettes on YouTube

Chuan Luo[1], Xiaolong Zheng[1,2], Daniel Dajun Zeng[1,3], Scott Leischow[4],
Kainan Cui[1,5], Zhu Zhang[1], and Saike He[1]

[1] The State Key Laboratory of Management and Control for Complex Systems,
Institute of Automation, Chinese Academy of Sciences, Beijing, China
[2] Dongguan Research Institute of CASIA,
Cloud Computing Center, Chinese Academy of Sciences, Dongguan, China
[3] Department of Management Information Systems,
The University of Arizona, Tucson, USA
[4] Mayo Clinic in Arizona, Phoenix, USA
[5] The School of Electronic and Information Engisneering,
Xi'an Jiaotong University, China
{chuan.luo,xiaolong.zheng,dajun.zeng,zhu.zhang,
saike.he}@ia.ac.cn, Leischow.Scott@mayo.edu, kainan.cui@live.cn

Abstract. Despite the growing number of videos featuring electronic cigarettes, there has been no investigation of the portrayal of these videos. This paper presents the first surveillance data of electronic cigarette videos on YouTube. Our results suggest that viewers are primarily being exposed to content promoting the use of these emerging tobacco products and the viewership is global. This study shows that it is critical to develop appropriate health campaigns to inform potential consumers of harms associated with electronic cigarette use.

Keywords: Electronic Cigarettes, YouTube, Data Mining, Public Health.

1 Introduction

Recent years have witnessed tremendous growth in the electronic cigarette marketplace. Electronic cigarettes are marketed online with testimonials from people trying to quit, despite the fact that electronic cigarettes are not scientifically proven or FDA-approved cessation aids [1]. There is a notable lack of public education dedicated to informing consumers about the health and safety concerns associated with electronic cigarettes [2]. However, there are many publicly available videos that purposely promote tobacco use on YouTube [3], [4]. Messages embedded in YouTube have the potential to influence tobacco-related attitudes, beliefs and behaviors [5]. Social media websites like YouTube have recently become a critical platform for health surveillance [6] and social intelligence [7].

Taking YouTube as a data source, previous researchers have studied information on 'smoking' [8], smoking cessation [9], smoking imagery associated with cigarettes [10], smokeless tobacco [11] and little cigars [12]. Although there is a study which mined data on usage of electronic cigarettes from YouTube videos [13], they didn't examine the portrayal of electronic cigarette contents.

D. Zeng et al. (Eds.): ICSH 2013, LNCS 8040, pp. 1–6, 2013.

Despite the growing literature on the portrayal of tobacco on YouTube, there are no published studies to date that have systematically assessed electronic cigarette content on YouTube. Given the potential that YouTube has to promote electronic cigarette use through user-generated content or covert advertising, this study aims to gain a better understanding of what electronic cigarette messages people are being exposed to on YouTube.

2   Methods

We first created a sample dataset from YouTube and then categorized these collected videos. The detailed information of each stage is described as follows.

2.1   Data Collection

We sampled electronic cigarette related videos on YouTube for study purpose in line with several previous related studies [8], [11], [12]. Using YouTube's search engine we conducted searches for electronic cigarette videos on February 3, 2013. The sample of YouTube videos for this study was selected from the top search results for the following search terms: "electronic cigarettes", "e-cigarettes", "ecigarettes", "ecigs", "smoking electronic cigarettes", "smoking e-cigarettes", "smoking ecigarettes", "smoking ecigs". These eight search terms were chosen because they are the most frequently used terms for electronic cigarettes and they can cover both "pro" and "anti" electronic cigarette videos, hopefully. In addition, through a Google Trends [14] analysis we found that there is a higher proportion of web traffic searching for these search terms than other electronic cigarette terms.

Two searches were conducted for each term (a) "by relevance" and (b) "by view count". These two kinds of search strategy were chosen to mimic the typical user behavior by using the default search strategy (searching "by relevance") as well as capture the most popular videos (searching "by view count").

Based on insight on user browsing behavior gained from previous studies [15] on a several Internet search engines indicating that the majority of people will only click on the first page of search results, we assume that few users would watch more than 20 videos since the first page of YouTube search results contains 20 videos. As a result, the sample was limited to the top 20 videos for each search. The initial sample included 320 videos in total (20 videos for each of the eight search terms and each of the two search strategies).

After obtaining the initial sample for this study from the first stage, we then eliminated videos that were not relevant to electronic cigarettes and videos that were duplicates. Videos were considered not relevant to electronic cigarettes if they didn't feature electronic cigarettes or there was only a brief mention or image of electronic cigarettes. Duplicate videos that appeared more than once by using different search terms and search strategies were also eliminated from the initial sample.

In the end, we obtained a total of 196 unique electronic cigarette related YouTube videos that were coded and analyzed in later stages to achieve the research goal of this study.

2.2   Video Coding

To access the overall portrayal of these electronic cigarette YouTube videos, we first rated the videos on whether they had contents that were "pro", "anti" or "neutral" to electronic cigarettes. "Pro" was defined as promoting the use of electronic cigarettes, such as presenting the advantage of electronic cigarettes, sharing their using experience with positive attitude toward electronic cigarettes, or making them look enjoyable or socially acceptable. Videos about quitting, negative consequences of using electronic cigarettes, or those that contained obvious negative feedbacks or warnings were considered "anti" to electronic cigarettes. Any videos that were not easily classified as either "pro" or "anti", but included mention about electronic cigarettes, were rated as "neutral" because they could make electronic cigarettes appear either positive or negative depending on the perspective of the video viewer when he/she was watching.

Within each portrayal category, videos were further classified by genre of YouTube video. The genres include advertisement, user sharing, product review, introduction, celebrity use, free trial, news clip and other TV program. These genres were chosen based on recurring themes in the 196 videos. Detailed description of each genre is shown as follows.

Table 1. Description of each genre

Genre	Description
Advertisement	Videos created by companies to promote a specific brand or product
User sharing	Videos uploaded by users to share experience or tips
Product review	Videos comparing multiple different products
Introduction	Videos introducing electronic cigarettes in general
Celebrity use	Videos showing several celebrities used electronic cigarettes
Free trial	Videos featuring URL links or store address to get free products
News clip	News clips reporting electronic cigarettes
Other TV program	Including TV shows, interviews which focused on electronic cigarettes

Finally, to perform the later video analysis, basic information was collected from each of the YouTube videos, including the video title, the username of person uploading the video, the number of views, favorites, likes and dislikes since YouTube users can archive videos by labeling a video as a "favorite" one and rate videos by whether they "like" or "dislike" a video. Given that YouTube has made several demographic information available, we also documented the countries in which the video was most frequently watched, age (13-17, 18-24, 25-34, 35-44, 45-54, 55-64), and gender of those most likely to watch the video.

3   Results

Among all the sample videos, 94% (n=185) were "pro" electronic cigarettes and 4% (n=8) were neutral, while there were only 2% (n=3) were "anti" electronic cigarettes. Obviously, the vast majority of the videos promoted the use of electronic cigarettes.

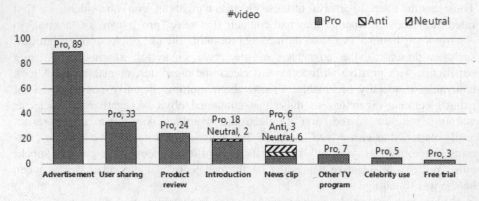

Fig. 1. Genres of YouTube videos

The distribution of video amount over the 8 genres is presented in the above Figure 1. Among all the "pro" videos, 48.1% (n=89) were advertisement. All the user sharing videos (n=33) were "pro" ones. In the news clip genre, there were 6 videos which promoted electronic cigarettes. The 3 "anti" videos were all news clips.

The following Table 2 shows the video statistics associated with the "pro", "anti" and "neutral" videos, which reflects the degree of viewer active participation.

Table 2. Video statistics associated with YouTube videos

		"pro" (n=185)	"anti" (n=3)	"neutral" (n=8)
#view	Total	**14,335,197**	174,638	324,486
	Average	77,488	58,213	40,561
	Range	2-2,362,588	284-90,060	8-122,256
#comment	Total	14,746	1,080	257
	Average	81	**360**	37
	Range	0-2,148	0-841	0-206
#favorite	Total	8,540	24	122
	Average	**56**	12	20
	Range	0-682	0-24	0-80
#like	Total	24,092	102	234
	Average	**135**	34	33
	Range	0-4,430	0-58	0-133
#dislike	Total	3,158	886	58
	Average	18	**295**	8
	Range	0-582	0-871	0-48

The 185 "pro" videos had been watched by 14,335,197 times in total and it had 56 "favorites" and 135 "likes" averagely, which were higher than "anti" and "neutral" videos. On the other hand, it had 295 "dislikes" and 360 comments for "anti" videos averagely that were much higher than "pro" videos. Preliminary examination showed that most of the comments were explicitly against the opinion that electronic cigarettes were negative for public health. In one word, "pro" electronic cigarette views are dominated the discussion on YouTube.

According to the demographic information available on YouTube, the majority of the audience was from the "Male, 45-54 years" group. In terms of the nationality of the audience, Figure 2 has shown the number of videos for each country, in which the video was popular.

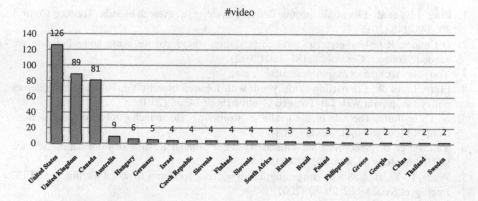

Fig. 2. Country of the majority of audience (top 3 countries for each video are available)

It is clear the viewership of these electronic cigarette videos is global. However, most videos were popular in United States, United Kingdom and Canada. This result reflects the fact that people in these countries are particularly interested in electronic cigarettes and marketers are putting many promotional efforts in these countries.

4   Discussion and Conclusion

To the best of our knowledge, this is one of the first studies to document the quantity, portrayal and reach of electronic cigarette videos on YouTube. The vast majority of information on YouTube about electronic cigarettes promotes their use. In addition, "pro" electronic cigarette views are dominated the discussion on YouTube, while "anti" electronic cigarette voice are so weak.

Our results have several implications regarding policy making. First, it's urgent to monitor electronic cigarette videos posted on YouTube and other social media websites. Second, public health organizations should appropriately inform potential consumers of harms associated with electronic cigarette use. Third, governments may consider developing health messages to counter "pro" electronic cigarette content on YouTube.

The results presented in our study highlight the extent of "pro" electronic cigarette contents on YouTube. It is critical to develop appropriate health campaigns to inform potential consumers of harms associated with electronic cigarette use. Further research is needed to evaluate the influence of electronic cigarette contents on people.

Acknowledgments. This work is partially funded through NNSFC Grants #71025001, #71103180, #91124001, #91024030, and 91124002, MOH Grants #2013ZX10004218 and #2012ZX10004801.

References

1. Etter, J.F., et al.: Electronic nicotine delivery systems: a research agenda. Tobacco Control 20, 243–248 (2011)
2. O'Connor, R.J.: Non-cigarette tobacco products: what have we learnt and where are we headed? Tobacco Control 21, 181–190 (2012)
3. YouTube, https://www.youtube.com/
4. Elkin, L., et al.: Connecting world youth with tobacco brands: YouTube and the internet policy vacuum on Web 2.0. Tobacco Control 19, 361–366 (2010)
5. N. C. Institute, The role of the media in promoting and reducing tobacco use. Tobacco Control Monograph, Bethesda (2008)
6. Yan, P., et al.: Syndromic surveillance systems. Annual Review of Information Science and Technology 42, 425–495 (2008)
7. Wang, F.-Y., et al.: Social computing: From social informatics to social intelligence. IEEE Intelligent Systems 22, 79–83 (2007)
8. Freeman, B., Chapman, S.: Is "YouTube" telling or selling you something? Tobacco content on the YouTube video-sharing website. Tobacco Control 16, 207–210 (2007)
9. Backinger, C.L., et al.: YouTube as a source of quitting smoking information. Tobacco Control 20, 119–122 (2011)
10. Forsyth, S.R., Malone, R.E.: "I'll be your cigarette–light me up and get on with it": examining smoking imagery on YouTube. Nicotine & Tobacco Research 12, 810–816 (2010)
11. Bromberg, J.E., et al.: Portrayal of Smokeless Tobacco in YouTube Videos. Nicotine & Tobacco Research 14, 455–462 (2012)
12. Richardson, A., Vallone, D.M.: YouTube: a promotional vehicle for little cigars and cigarillos? Tobacco Control (October 9, 2012)
13. Hua, M., et al.: Mining data on usage of electronic nicotine delivery systems (ENDS) from YouTube videos. Tobacco Control 22, 103–106 (2013)
14. Google Trends, http://www.google.com/trends/
15. Jansen, B.J., Spink, A.: How are we searching the world wide web?: a comparison of nine search engine transaction logs. Inf. Process. Manage. 42, 248–263 (2006)

The Effectiveness of Smoking Cessation Intervention on Facebook: A Preliminary Study of Posts and Users

Mi Zhang and Christopher C. Yang

College of Information Science and Technology, Drexel University, Philadelphia, PA
{mi.zhang,chris.yang}@drexel.edu

Abstract. Smoking causes many serious illnesses such as lung cancer, chronic bronchitis, and emphysem. Some intervention programs of smoking cessation are developed online, which can reach a large number of people at any time. QuitNet is one of the most popular websites of smoking cessation. It developed a public page on Facebook, providing information and initiating discussions on smoking cessation. In this study, we explore the features of QuitNet Facebook through preliminary qualitative and quantitative analysis. We collect data of posts and comments from 04/01/2011 to 06/31/2011on QuitNet Facebook and analyze the data from the post and user perspectives. For the post perspective, we analyze popular posts which receive the most and the soonest comments from Facebook users, and find that most of these posts ask for responses of user motivations, methods, experiences and emotions of smoking abstinence. For the user perspective, we analyze users who make comments more frequently and immediately after a post being published, and find that users at the maintenance stage of smoking cessation are more active than those at the early actions stage.

Keywords: QuitNet, Facebook, Smoking Cessation, Social Media, Health 2.0.

1   Introduction

Internet is an important resource for people to seek for health information. A report in 2009 showed that 61% of American adults went online to look for health information [1]. Internet use has both direct and indirect relations to subjective health [2]. With the development of Web 2.0, a related concept – Health 2.0 emerged, of which social networking is an important feature [3], [4]. Many online communities and social networking groups are developed for people to discuss health issues and interact with each other. Fox et al. reported that "the social life of health information is robust", with the fact that 52% online health inquired involved interaction with others [1]. Generally, there are two types of online communities for healthcare communication. Some communities or forums are developed solely for health issues, like MedHelp[1], patientslikeme[2], and forums for specific health problems; The other type of health communities are developed on popular online social media sites, including Facebook,

---

[1] http://www.medhelp.org/
[2] http://www.patientslikeme.com

D. Zeng et al. (Eds.): ICSH 2013, LNCS 8040, pp. 7–17, 2013.

Twitter, LinkedIn, Blogs, YouTube, Second Life, etc [5]. A recent research reported that, comparing to online support groups and blogs, social networking sites like MySpace and Facebook can attract more users, and has the potential to reach the target population regardless of socioeconomic and health-related characteristics [6].

Smoking causes the death of 440,000 U.S. citizens every year [7]. It is associated with cancers of more than ten organs. Lung diseases and heart diseases are especially highly related with tobacco use. Although the proportion of U.S. adult smokers declined in recent years, more than 20% of U.S. adults still smoked cigarettes in 2008 [8]. Many intervention programs are developed for smoking cessation. In recent years, online smoking cessation intervention programs attract increasing attention, because they can reach a large number of people at different locations. QuitNet[3] is one of the most popular websites for smoking cessation in United States. It provides different services to help users quit smoking, including online communities for user interactions. A lot of research investigates features of QuitNet and other smoking cessation websites. It is found that active participants in online intervention programs tend to be female, older and abstinent of smoking [9], [10]. People participating in support communities are more likely to be continuously abstinent [9], [11]. Web-based, tailored, and interactive smoking cessation interventions are more effective [12]. There are four key areas of online smoking cessation resources: cessation, prevention, social support and professional development and training [13]. Compared to earlier programs, present online smoking cessation interventions focus more on providing advice to quit, practical counseling, and enhancing motivation to quit smoking through personal relevance and risks [14].

Besides specific online communities for smoking cessation, there are also communities developed on popular social media sites such as MySpace, Facebook and Twitter. QuitNet built a public page on Facebook[4], which is the most popular social networking website. As the second-top website in the world [15], Facebook attracts more than 600 million daily active users [16]. Different groups and communities are built on Facebook. The average Facebook user is connected to 80 community pages, groups and events. The public page of QuitNet on Facebook was built on 2009. Every registered Facebook user can browse the page. Users who "like" this page could receive information from QuitNet directly and participate in the discussions. The QuitNet Facebook page provides a tremendous opportunity to reach a large number of potential users for smoking cessation intervention. However, there are few studies investigating this particular communication channel for smoking cessation. There are also public pages and discussion groups on Facebook for other health topics. Posts from 15 groups of diabetes on Facebook were analyzed in a study. It was found that patients with diabetes used Facebook to share personal information, to request guidance and feedback for the disease, and to receive emotional support [17]. In another study, 620 breast cancer groups on Facebook were investigated, which found that the main purposes of these groups were fundraising, awareness, product or service promotion, and patient/caregiver support [18]. There are also

---

[3] http://www.quitnet.com/qnhomepage.aspx
[4] https://www.facebook.com/QuitNet

groups for concussion (brain injury) on Facebook. Three meaningful purposes of posts of these groups are relating personal experience, seeking explicit information, and offering explicit advice [19]. In this study, we will focus on the public page of smoking cessation built by QuitNet on Facebook.

QuitNet Facebook and QuitNet Forum on its original website represent two different types of online health communities mentioned above. Users of QuitNet Forum participate in the community solely for smoking cessation issues. They take some efforts to log in (with a user name and password) and actively acquire smoking cessation information. But QuitNet Facebook is built on a popular social networking site, and most of its users are connected to Facebook regularly for different social purposes, not specifically for smoking cessation. When QuitNet Facebook publishes a new post, the information would be sent to its users' Facebook "news feeds". So the users receive the quit information "passively" in real time, and they do not need to take additional efforts to join a specific community of smoking cessation. In this way, they could participate in the discussions of smoking quitting, while taking part in other regular social activities on Facebook. Our earlier research showed that QuitNet on Facebook could attract users with a wider range of smoking statuses than QuitNet Forum [20]. As QuitNet Facebook is more convenient for people to receive information about smoking cessation and participate in the discussions, it is anticipated that people could respond to a post on QuitNet Facebook much faster than that on specific online smoking cessation forums. Currently, only the page admin could start a new post on QuitNet Facebook. Facebook users who like the page can respond to each post and make comments. In this study, we analyze the number of responses and response immediacy to a post of QuitNet Facebook users. Our proposed research questions are based on two perspectives:

1. Post perspective: what kinds of posts receive the most frequent and the soonest responses from Facebook users?
2. User Perspective: what kinds of users respond more frequently and immediately to posts from QuitNet Facebook?

2   Methods

We collect a three-month dataset between 04/01/2011 and 06/31/2011 from the public page of QuitNet on Facebook, including posts during that period and all the comments of them. There are 111 posts, 2578 comments and 664 users extracted.

To answer the first research question, we calculate the comment quantity and the first response time for each post. The comment quantity is the total number of comments received by a post, and the first response time is after how many seconds that the post receives the first comment since it is published. The two indicators reflect the frequency and immediacy that a post attracts users' attention. The relation of the comment quantity and the first response time is analyzed using Spearman's correlation analysis. The content of posts with the highest comment quantity and the lowest first response time is analyzed.

For the second research question, quit status is introduced as a user characteristic, which is defined as the number of days that a former smoker has been abstinent from the day he stopped smoking to the day he posted the last message on QuitNet Facebook during the period of the dataset [20]. As an important characteristic of smoking quitters, quit status is also an indicator to measure the output of smoking cessation. On every Friday, QuitNet launches a post on Facebook, calling for people to report for how many days that they are abstinent of smoking. According to their replies in our dataset, we could calculate the quit statuses of some users. 394 users with available quit statuses are extracted. The comment quantity and the average response time of each of these users are calculated. The comment quantity of a user indicates the total number of comments he made on all the posts in the dataset. It could reflect the frequency that a user participates in discussions on QuitNet Facebook. For each user, we select all the posts that he has responded to, and extracts his first comment for each post to calculate the response time (note that a user may make multiple comments on the same post). The average value of response time to all posts is calculated, which is defined as the average response time of a user in this study. The average response time could reflect how soon a user responds to a post on average when taking part in a discussion on QuitNet Facebook. When analyzing the average response time of 394 users, four outliers are found. We remove these outliers and retain 390 users for later analysis. In our study, we first describe the statistics of all users' comment quantity and average response time, then the relations of quit status with comment quantity and average response time are analyzed. Spearman's correlation analysis is used. Usually, a smoking quitter moves five stages to quit smoking, which are precontemplation, contemplation, preparation, action and maintenance [21]. Action is the period that people take real actions to quit smoking. It includes an early action period of 0 to 3 month, and a late action period of 3 to 6 month after abstinence. Maintenance is the period beginning 6 months after action starts. Velicer etc. recommended 6 to 60 months as the duration of the maintenance stage [21]. In our study, users are categorized into five groups according to their quit statuses. The first group is composed by users at the early action stage of smoking cessation who have been abstinent for 0 to 90 days; the second group is composed by users at the late action stage who have been abstinent for 91 to 180 days; the third group is consisted of users at the early maintenance stage abstinent for 181 to 720 days; the fourth group is composed by users at the late maintenance stage who have been abstinent for 721 to 1800 days; and the fifth group is consisted of users who have been abstinent for more than 1800 days [20]. ANOVA with LSD post-hoc tests is carried out to compare comment quantity and average response time between users in different groups of quit statuses. SPSS 19 is used for all the analysis in our study.

3   Results

3.1   Post Perspective

There are 2578 comments made on the 111 posts in our dataset. Four posts do not have any comments. For the 107 posts which have at least one comment, the statistics of the comment quantity and the first response time is shown in Table 1.

Table 1. Statistics of Comment Quantity and First Response Time of Posts

	Mean	Median	Std. Deviation	Minimum	Maximum
Comment Amount	24.09	15.00	22.909	1	91
First Response Time (seconds)	1965.61	177.00	8663.521	91	81512

For the 107 posts, Spearman's correlation analysis shows a significant correlation between the comment quantity and the first response time (p<.001 and r=-.755).

On Fridays, QuitNet launches posts with the same content that "It's Friday --- Shout Your Stats". They receive the largest number of comments and the soonest responses. The top 10 posts with the highest comment quantity and the lowest first response time are shown in Table 2.

Table 2. Top 10 Posts With the Highest Comment Quantity and Lowest First Response Time

	Top 10 with largest comment quantity	Top 10 with lowest first response time
It's Friday -- Shout Your Stats!	X	X
How did you quit smoking? Did you go with NRT, Zyban, Chantix, an alternative method such as hypnosis/laser/acupuncture or Cold Turkey?	X	X
At what point in your quit did you feel as though you'd really quit for good?	X	
Happy Thursday! Name 3 things you LOVE about being a nonsmoker!	X	
What has meant the most to you about your quit?	X	X
There are so many bonuses to quitting, including better health and more money. What have you treated yourself to since you quit?	X	
What song best describes your quit?!	X	
At what point in your quit did you feel as though you had "turned a corner"?	X	X
Did you have a secret stash of smokes? If so, where did you hide your stash?	X	
What 1 word described you before your quit and what word would you use to describe yourself now?	X	
Many of us used tobacco as a reward. How do we reward ourselves without it?		X
Ask a kid under the age of 10 what they think about cigarettes and smoking.		X
What (or who) helps keep your quit going strong?!		X
What's the best advice on quitting you've ever received?		X
Smile and KTQ! Smoking wreaks havoc on your oral health and teeth.		X
What do you think? Should tobacco companies pay hospitals for costs relating to treating sick smokers? http://www.foxbusiness.com/market s/2011/04/29/jury-finds-tobacco-cos-responsible-smokers-health-costs/		X

3.2   User Perspective

For the 390 users, the range of their comment quantity is [1, 89], the mean is 5.28, and the standard deviation of 8.26. Their average response time covers a wide range, which is (29, 174337) (seconds). The mean of each user's average response time is 16993.54 (seconds), nearly 5 hours. We categorize users into seven groups according to their average response time. The distribution is shown in Table 3 and Figure 1.

Spearman's correlation analysis indicates significant correlation between user comment quantity and the average response time, with $p<.001$ and $r=.232$. ANOVA test with LSD post-hoc test is carried out to compare the means of comment quantity between different time groups as shown in Table 4, and the $p=.007$.

Table 3. User Groups Based on Average Response Time

	<600" (10 minutes)	601"-1800" (30 minutes)	1801"-3600" (1 hour)	3601"-7200" (2 hours)	7201" – 18000" (5 hours)	18001"-86400" (1 day)	>86400" (1 day)
# of users	52	57	58	56	73	74	20
Percentage	13.3%	14.6%	14.9%	14.4%	18.7%	19.0%	5.1%

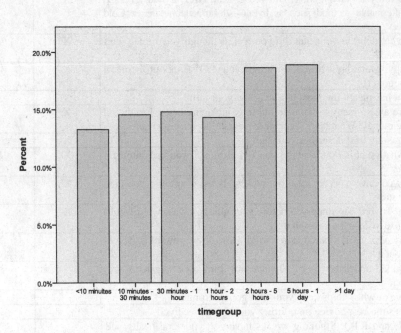

Fig. 1. User Distribution Across Time Groups

Table 4. Statistics of User Comment Quantity of Different Time Groups

	Mean	Std. Deviation
<600'' (10 minutes)	1.96	1.76
601''-1800'' (30 minutes)	3.98	6.03
1801''-3600'' (1 hour)	5.38	5.24
3601''-7200'' (2 hours)	4.61	5.76
7201'' – 18000'' (5 hours)	7.18	11.76
18001''-86400'' (1 day)	7.01	11.03
> 86400'' (1 day)	5.95	7.09

Spearman's correlation analysis shows no correlation between user quit status and the comment quantity with p=.982. However, there is significant negative correlation between quit status and the average response time with p=.017 and r=-.121. Users are categorized into five groups of different quit statuses. The statistics of comment quantity and average response time for users in each group are shown in Table 5.

Table 5. Statistics of Comment Quantity and Average Response Time of Different Quit Status Groups

Quit status (days)	N	Comment Number		Average Response Time	
		Mean	Std. deviation	Mean	Std. deviation
0-90	97	3.86	4.352	23060.45	37206.170
91-180	78	5.76	6.186	15830.18	23476.652
181-720	114	5.61	7.713	15650.40	31534.693
721-1800	69	6.96	14.258	13844.94	31345.079
>1800	32	3.72	4.946	13013.00	18179.737

The p values for ANOVA tests of comment quantity and average response time between the five groups are all above 0.1. But in LSD post-hoc tests, for group 1 and group 4, and group 4 and group 5, the p values for comment quantity are below 0.1; and for group 1 & group 3, and group 1 & group 4, the p values for average response time are below 0.1.

4 Discussions

4.1 Post Perspective

For a post on QuitNet Facebook, its comment quantity reflects how many people are attracted to take part in the discussion, and the first response time reflects how soon it attracts people's attention. Both of them are indicators to measure whether people are interested in the post. Comment quantity and the first response time to a post are negatively correlated, which means that posts which attract more people also tend to attract them faster. So a post which arouses great interests of users would have a large number of comments and fast response time.

According to Table 2, posts with a large number of comments all ask for people's responses. Some of them ask people to share their experiences and emotions during abstinence period, and others discuss motivations and methods of smoking cessation. Most posts with low first response time contain fewer words. With a large amount of information on Facebook, short posts are easier to attract people. When users take part in the discussion of a post, they usually read other's replies as well. So it is important for QuitNet Facebook to publish posts with interesting topics and contents which could attract people to participate in and interact with others. In this way, people could learn from each other about motivations and methods to quit smoking. At the same time, sharing experiences and emotions could provide emotional supports for each other as well.

Posts with few comments and slow response usually have long contents. Most of them provide information of smoking cessation and do not ask for user responses. Some of them simply link to a long article in other websites. Posts with long messages could not draw users' attention because typical Facebook messages are concise. Users do not tend to take extended time to respond to long messages.

4.2   User Perspective

On average, most users respond to a post within 24 hours after the post is published by QuitNet Facebook. The mean of user average response time is nearly 5 hours, and the range is wide. The seven user groups in Table 3 and Figure 1 reflect the levels of their response speed on average. From the first group to the last group, users respectively respond to a post within 10 minutes, 30 minutes, 1 hour, 2 hours, 5hours, 1 day and after 1day on average. The first six groups contain similar numbers of users, which means that users are equally distributed in groups within one day. So, there is no particular tendency of user average response time within one day, and their response behaviors vary greatly.

There is significantly positive correlation between user comment quantity and average response time. From Table 4, users with the average response time below 10 minutes only publish less than two comments on average. Among the 52 users who respond to a post within 10 minutes, 33 of them only comment once in our dataset. So, in the first group in Table 4, most users are not active to participate in the QuitNet Facebook. The reason for their participations may be that the posts from QuitNet Facebook appear at the beginning of their Facebook news feeds by chance. They reply them inadvertently and the response time is fast. If the posts of QuitNet appear at the end of their Facebook news feeds, they may or may not reply any more. Users with average response time from 2 hours to 1 day frequently make comments. They actively participate in discussions of QuitNet Facebook and reply to a large number of posts.

Although no correlation is found between user quit status and comment quantity, there is a slight negative correlation between quit status and the average response time. Recent smoking quitters with a short abstinence time tend to respond to posts slowly. Especially, users at maintenance stage of smoking cessation (group 3 and group 4 in Table 5) significantly respond faster than users at the early action stage (group 1 in Table 5). According to post-hoc tests of ANOVA on comment quantity, users at late maintenance stage (group 4 in Table 5) make more comments than users at early action stage (group 1 in Table 5). In our former study [20], we also found that users at early maintenance stage (group 3 in Table 5) have significantly higher degrees than users in group 1 in a social network built on user interactions in the same dataset. Based on all the evidences above, it could be concluded that on QuitNet Facebook, people who have been abstinent for a relatively long time and at the maintenance stage perform more actively than users who just start to take actions to quit smoking. There are two possible reasons to explain this phenomenon. First, people at the early stage of smoking cessation usually need more professional help. They may go to medical institute for consulting. Even if they use Internet to seek for information, they are more likely to go to professional websites of smoking cessation, but not popular social networking sites. However, people who have finished action stage and at the maintenance of abstinence may not need medical or professional support any more. But they still concern the topic of quitting smoking. So they "like" QuitNet page on Facebook. When they go to Facebook for social networking in their daily life, they casually take part in some informal discussions about quitting smoking. Second, many posts of QuitNet Facebook ask questions about experiences of smoking cessation, as well as motivations and methods to quit. People at the early action stage may not have enough experiences to share, so they feel difficult to answer these questions and take part in the interactions. But for people at the maintenance stage, they already have rich experiences and are able to answer these questions. They might introduce their methods, motivations, and experiences to quit smoking, and provide supports for others.

5   Conclusion

In this study, we analyzed QuitNet Facebook from the perspectives of post and user respectively. For the post perspective, we explored the features of popular posts which received a large number of comments and fast responses. It is found that the comment quantity of posts and the first response time to posts are negatively correlated. Most popular posts ask for responses from users about their motivations, methods, experiences and emotions during smoking cessation, and contain only a few words. For the user perspective, we explored the relations between quit status, comment quantity and average response time. We found that users at the maintenance stage of smoking cessation respond more frequently and faster than users at the early action stage. The limitations for this study include: (1) the quit statuses of users may not be accurate because they are calculated based on user self-reported online comments; (2) the dataset only includes data of three months, but the contents and features of posts may vary in different periods; (3) we did not apply detailed qualitative analysis on post contents, so the result and discussion are not specific. In the future study, we plan to collect new dataset and adopt different methods like survey to get user characteristics. We will also implement qualitative analysis on posts and comments to investigate user behaviors in detail. Smoking cessation programs based on public social networking sites provide a new way to support people to quit smoking. Understanding the features of these programs could help us provide better supports and services to achieve the best effects.

References

1. Fox, S., Jones, S.: The Social Life of Health Information, http://www.pewinternet.org/~/media//Files/Reports/2009/PIP_Health_2009.pdf
2. Wangberg, S.C., Andreassen, H.K., Prokosch, H.U., Santana, S.M., Sørensen, T., Chronaki, C.E.: Relations Between Internet Use, Socio-economic Status (SES), Social Support and Subjective Health. Health Promotion International 23, 70–78 (2008)
3. Eysenbach, G.: Medicine 2.0: Social Networking, Collaboration, Participation, Apomediation, and Openness. Journal of Medical Internet Research 10, e22 (2008)
4. VanDeBelt, T.H., Engelen, L., Berben, S., Schoonhoven, L.: Definition of Health 2.0 and Medicine 2.0: a Systematic Review. Journal of Medical Internet Research 12, e18 (2012)
5. Backman, C., Dolack, S., Dunyak, D., Lutz, L., Tegen, A., Warner, D., Wieland, L.: Social Media + Healthcare, http://library.ahima.org/xpedio/groups/public/documents/ahima/bok1_048693.hcsp?dDocName=bok1_0
6. Chou, W.S., Hunt, Y.M., Beckjord, E.B., Moser, R.P., Hesse, B.W.: Social Media Use in the United States: Implications for Health Communication. Journal of Medical Internet Research 11, e48 (2009)
7. National Institute of Drug Abuse: What are the Medical Consequences of Tobacco Use? http://www.drugabuse.gov/publications/research-reports/tobacco-addiction/what-are-medical-consequences-tobacco-use
8. Centers for Disease Control and Prevention: Cigarette Smoking Among Adults and Trends in Smoking Cessation, http://www.cdc.gov/mmwr/preview/mmwrhtml/mm5844a2.htm
9. An, L.C., Schillo, B.A., Saul, J.E., Wendling, A.H., Klatt, C.M., Berg, C.J., Ahulwalia, J.S., Kavanaugh, A.M., Christenson, M., Luxenberg, M.G.: Utilization of smoking cessation informational, interactive, and online community resources as predictors of abstinence: cohort study. Journal of Medical Internet Research 10, e55 (2008)
10. Cobb, N.K., Graham, A.L.: Characterizing Internet searchers of smoking cessation information. Journal of Medical Internet Research 8, e17 (2006)
11. Cobb, N.K., Graham, A.L., Bock, B.C., Papandonatos, G., Abrams, D.B.: Initial evaluation of a real-world Internet smoking cessation system. Nicotine Tob. Res. 7, 201–216 (2005)
12. Shahab, L., McEwen, A.: Online support for smoking cessation: a systematic review of the literature. Addiction 104, 1792–1804 (2009)
13. Norman, C.D., McIntosh, S., Selby, P., Eysenbach, G.: Web-assisted tobacco interventions: empowering change in the global fight for the public's (e)health. Journal of Medical Internet Research 10, e48 (2008)
14. Bock, B.C., Graham, A.L., Whiteley, J.A., Stoddard, J.L.: A review of web-assisted tobacco interventions (WATIs). Journal of Medical Internet Research 10, e39 (2008)
15. Alexa: Top Sites, http://www.alexa.com/topsites
16. Facebook: Facebook Statistics, http://newsroom.fb.com/Key-Facts
17. Greene, J.A., Choudhry, N.K., Kilabuk, E., Shrank, W.H.: Online Social Networking by Patients with Diabetes: a Qualitative Evaluation of Communication with Facebook. Journal of General Internal Medicine 26, 287–292 (2010)

18. Bender, J.L., Jimenez-Marroquin, M.C., Jadad, A.R.: Seeking Support on Facebook: a Content Analysis of Breast Cancer Groups. Journal of Medical Internet Research 13, e16 (2011)
19. Ahmed, O.H., Sullivan, S.J., Schneiders, A.G., Mccrory, P.: iSupport: Do Social Networking Sites Have a Role to Play in Concussion Awareness? Disability and Rehabilitation 32, 1877–1883 (2010)
20. Zhang, M., Yang, C.C., Li, J.: A Comparative Study of Smoking Cessation Intervention Programs on Social Media. In: Yang, S.J., Greenberg, A.M., Endsley, M. (eds.) SBP 2012. LNCS, vol. 7227, pp. 87–96. Springer, Heidelberg (2012)
21. Velicer, W.F., Prochaska, J.O., Rossi, J.S., Snow, M.: Assessing Outcome in Smoking Cessation Studies. Psychological Bulletin 111, 23–41 (1992)

An Empirical Analysis of Social Interaction on Tobacco-Oriented Social Networks

Yunji Liang[1,2], Xiaolong Zheng[3,4], Daniel Dajun Zeng[2,3,*], Xingshe Zhou[1,*], and Scott Leischow[5]

[1] School of Computer Science, Northwestern Polytechnical University, Xi'an, China
[2] Department of Management Information System,
University of Arizona, Tucson, Arizona, USA
[3] The State Key Laboratory of Management and Control for Complex Systems,
Institute of Automation, Chinese Academy of Sciences, Beijing, China
[4] Dongguan Research Institute of CASIA, Cloud Computing Center,
Chinese Academy of Sciences, Songshan Lake, Dongguan, China
[5] Mayo Clinic in Arizona, Phoenix, USA

Abstract. Social media is widely utilized in the tobacco control campaigns. It is a great challenge to evaluate the efficiency of tobacco control policies on social network sites and find gaps among tobacco-oriented social networks. In this paper, we construct three tobacco-oriented social networks according to user interaction on Facebook tobacco-related fan pages. We further investigate the interaction patterns including temporal distribution and interaction patterns to reveal the differences of tobacco-oriented social networks. Our empirical analysis demonstrates that: 1) the user interaction on the pro-tobacco fan pages is more active. Fan pages for tobacco promotion are more successful in obtaining more user attention. 2) The gap between tobacco promotion and tobacco control is widening. These empirical results can provide us significant insights into understanding the evolutionary patterns of social interaction in tobacco-oriented social networks and further help the government departments of tobacco control to make reasonable decisions.

Keywords: Tobacco, User Interaction, Social Network, Facebook, Fan Page.

1   Introduction

Social Media such as Facebook, YouTube, and Twitter is becoming the battlefield of tobacco. Tobacco companies stand to benefit greatly from the marketing potential of social media, without themselves being at significant risk of being implicated in violating any laws [1], such as cigarette promotion on Facebook [2], pro-tobacco video clips on YouTube [1] and mobile applications ('ishisha' and 'Cigar Boss') for tobacco promotion. By contrast, as a primary source of health information for the general public, news coverage has been widely utilized in anti-tobacco campaigns to

---

* Corresponding authors.

D. Zeng et al. (Eds.): ICSH 2013, LNCS 8040, pp. 18–23, 2013.

raise public anti-tobacco awareness with horrible facts such as lung cancers and toxic chemicals derived from tobacco. In addition, for smokers, social media is adopted to kick the bad habit by tracking cigarette consumption and offering tobacco cessation assistance with social support such as QuitNet and EX [3, 4].

However, with the progression of new technology, it is a great challenge to quantify gaps among tobacco promotion, tobacco control and tobacco cessation forces on social media [5].There is a growing need for an active research to ensure that advocacy efforts have the desired effect to improve future campaigns and maximize impact [6]. The comparison of three forces on social media may help to find the gaps and loopholes, evaluate the efficiency of tobacco control policies in the new media environment. Furthermore, it provides solid and impressive proofs for the decision makers.

To address the above problem, in this paper, we investigate the social interaction on tobacco-oriented social networks. According to user interactions on Facebook tobacco-related fan pages, we extracted three tobacco-oriented social networks, named pro-tobacco, anti-tobacco and quitting-tobacco social network individually. Based on those three tobacco-oriented social networks, we conduct a comparative study of interaction patterns on tobacco-oriented social networks. The main contributions of the paper are two-folders: (1) To the best of our knowledge, it is the first time to provide large-scale tobacco-oriented social networks based on user interaction on social network; (2) We aim to find the gaps among different forces with the analysis of interaction of tobacco-oriented social networks.

The remainder of this paper is organized as follows. The data collection is presented in Section 2. In Section 3, we conduct a comparative analysis of user interaction including temporal distribution and interaction patterns. Section 4 concludes this paper and presents our future work as well.

2   Data Collection on Facebook Fan Pages

Facebook fan page is a public profile that enables users to share their business and products with Facebook users [2]. In this paper, we mainly focus on the interaction (post likes and comments) on Facebook tobacco-related fan pages. The data collection on Facebook consists of two steps: offline data preparation and online data collection.

Table 1. Keywords for Facebook searches

Keywords	tobacco, smoking, cigarette, anti-tobacco, anti-smoking, anti-cigarette, tobacco free, smoking free, cigarette free, quit smoking, stop smoking, smokeless, beedi, cigars, cigar, snuffs, hookah, pipe smoking, snuff, snus, quit cigarette, stop cigarette, quit tobacco, stop tobacco, tobacco addiction, smoking addiction, cigarette addiction, smoking cessation, tobacco cessation, cigarette cessation, nicotine, nicotine addiction, nicotine prevention, nicotine cessation

In the offline data preparation, we first conduct keyword searches for tobacco-related fan pages using the keywords shown in Table 1. Then, according to the profiles of fan pages, all retrieved fan pages are classified into 4 types by two coders manually: (0: unrelated to tobacco; 1: tobacco promotion; 2: tobacco control; 3: tobacco cessation). A third coder coded the fan pages for which there was no agreement between the first two coders. If the third coder disagreed with each of the first two coders, that fan pages are excluded.

For the online data collection, the basic information of fan pages is collected including the number of fan page likes, post volume and post content. More importantly, the user interaction records on Facebook fan pages are gathered as well. When a Facebook user A comments or likes a post launched by Facebook user B, it is regarded that user interaction occurs between A and B.

Totally, we got 2149 tobacco-related fan pages (708 for tobacco promotion, 684 for tobacco control and 757 for tobacco cessation). Specifically, 557 of the pro-tobacco fan pages are about tobacco brands (such as new port, camel and black devil), tobacco-related products such as smoking pipe, tobacco promotion information (such as free-duty cigarettes and cheap online tobacco shops) and protest for tobacco control. 151 of the pro-tobacco fan pages are concerned about electronic cigarettes. As shown in Table 2, the pro-tobacco group overwhelms other groups in terms of page likes, post like and comments.

Table 2. Overview of three tobacco-oriented fan pages

Group of Fan Pages	Page Volume	Page Like	Post Like	Comment
Tobacco Promotion	708	2909532	14660450	521091
Tobacco Control	684	1232153	489853	81236
Tobacco Cessation	757	1569490	837938	191004

3   Comparative Analysis of Interaction on Tobacco-Oriented Social Networks

To compare user interaction in the three groups, we analyze the temporal distribution of post volume, and interaction patterns including page likes, post volume and comments of the three tobacco-oriented social networks.

3.1   Temporal Distribution of Post Volume for Fan Pages

We analyze the temporal distribution of post volume on fan pages for different groups. As shown in Fig. 2, the post volumes of three groups have been increasing since 2008. The year of 2011 witnessed the breakthrough of the three groups with more than 1000 posts per month. The explosive growth happened at July, 2012 with rapid expansion of gap between pro-tobacco group and anti-tobacco group. Compared with the explosive growth for pro-tobacco and quitting tobacco groups, the anti-tobacco group experienced a steady growth. As time goes by, the gap between anti-tobacco and pro-tobacco has been widening. This indicates that we are facing with a tremendous challenge for tobacco control.

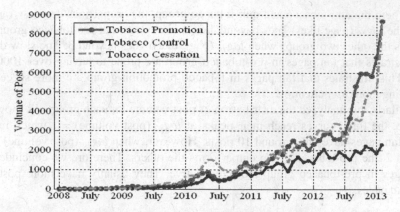

Fig. 1. Temporal distribution of the post volume on three tobacco-oriented groups

3.2 Interaction Patterns on Tobacco-Oriented Fan Pages

As shown in Fig. 2a, the number of page likes (measured by log_{10}) is presented on horizontal axis. While the value on vertical axis indicates the percentage of fan pages with the given page likes. According to Fig. 2a, the curves of anti-tobacco ecosystem and quitting-tobacco reach the peak at log_{10}(page likes) =1.5, which means most of fan pages in those two of groups have approximating $10^{1.5} \approx 32$ page likes. By contrast, for the pro-tobacco group, the curve peaks at log_{10} (page likes) = 3 with 21.6%. That means the 21.6% of pro-tobacco fan pages have approximating 10^3=1000 page likes.

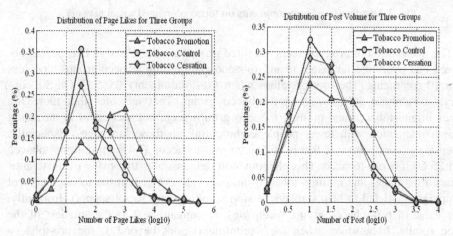

Fig. 2. (a) Distribution of page likes on three tobacco-oriented groups; (b) Distribution of post volume

22   Y. Liang et al.

For both the anti-tobacco and quit-tobacco group, the proportions decrease rapidly when the log_{10} (page likes) goes beyond 1.5. It is obvious that pro-tobacco group out weights the other two groups when log_{10} (page likes) goes beyond 3. The slow decay demonstrates that fan pages in pro-tobacco group are prone to having over 1000 fan likes. This illustrates that fan pages in tobacco promotion group are more successful in gaining more user attention.

Similarly, we analyzed the distribution of post volume for each group. As shown in Fig. 2b, the three curves reach their peaks at log_{10} (post volume) =1, which means many fan pages have only around 10 posts. However, when log_{10} (post volume) goes beyond 2, the pro-tobacco group outperforms the others. Therefore we conclude that fan pages in pro-tobacco group are more active. They usually have more posts on each fan pages.

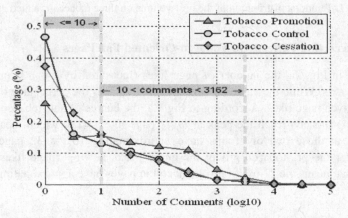

Fig. 3. Distribution of post comments on tobacco-oriented social networks

The distribution of post comments in three groups are illustrated in Fig. 3. It is observed that over 70% fan pages in anti-tobacco and quitting tobacco groups have less than 10 comments (The sum of values when log_{10} (comment)=0,0.5,1). On the contrary, it is about 56% for the pro-tobacco group. That indicates that more fan pages in anti-tobacco and quitting tobacco groups seem not successful in attracting human interaction with fewer people commenting on those fan pages. Especially, when log_{10} (comment) = 0, that is 46.5% for anti-tobacco, 37.4% for quitting tobacco and 25.6% for pro-tobacco. This phenomenon demonstrates that many of those anti-tobacco fan pages and quitting tobacco fan pages do not benefit the tobacco control campaigns, and fail to help smokers to stop smoking with social support. Ironically, that value of pro-tobacco group, when log_{10} (comment) = 0, is the smallest of the three results. Meanwhile, when log_{10} (comment) goes beyond 1, the pro-tobacco group out weights the other two groups. That means the comment interactions on pro-tobacco fan pages are more prosperous.

4   Conclusions

Social media is becoming the battlefield of tobacco-oriented war. However, how to quantify and evaluate the war forces is still a big challenge. In this paper, we first extract three large-scale tobacco-oriented social networks based user interaction on tobacco-related Facebook fan pages. Then a comparative study is conducted and reveals the differences of interaction patterns in the three social networks.

Based on the analysis of user interaction on tobacco-oriented social networks, we could draw the following conclusions: (1) compared with the pro-tobacco fan pages, lots of fan pages in anti-tobacco and quitting-tobacco groups are less effective with fewer posts, fewer comments and lower page likes; while pro-tobacco fan pages have succeed in attracting more potential users to involve or interact with the fan pages in pro-tobacco group; (2) There is a significant gap between pro-tobacco fan pages and anti-tobacco pages in term of post volume. And the gap is widening with the embracing of social media. We are now facing with a tremendous challenge for tobacco control.

Acknowledgements. This work was partially supported by the National Basic Research Program of China (No. 2012CB316400), the National Natural Science Foundation of China (No. 71103180, 91124001, 71025001, 91024030, 61222209 and 61103063), the Ministry of Health (No. 2012ZX10004801, 2013ZX10004218), the Program for New Century Excellent Talents in University (No. NCET-12-0466), the Specialized Research Fund for the Doctoral Program of Higher Education (No. 201261021100043), the Natural Science Basic Research Plan in Shaanxi Province of China (No. 2012JQ8028), and the Doctorate Foundation of Northwestern Polytechnical University.

References

1. Elkin, L., Thomson, G., Wilson, N.: Connecting world youth with tobacco brands: YouTube and the internet policy vacuum on Web 2.0. Tobacco Control 19, 361–366 (2010)
2. Freeman, B., Chapman, S.: British American Tobacco on Facebook: undermining article 13 of the global World Health Organization Framework Convention on Tobacco Control. Tobacco Control 19, 1–9 (2010)
3. Prochaska, J.J., Pechmann, C., Kim, R., Leonhardt, J.M.: Twitter=quitter? An analysis of Twitter quit smoking social networks. Tobobacco Control 21, 447–449 (2012)
4. Vallone, D.M., Duke, J.C., Mowery, P.D., et al.: The Impact of EX: Results from a Pilot Smoking-Cessation Media Campaign. American Journal of Preventive Medicine 38(3S), S312–S318 (2010)
5. Ribisl, K.M., Jo, C.: Tobacco control is losing ground in the web 2.0 era: invited commentary. Tobacco Control 21, 145–146 (2012)
6. How the news media influence tobacco use, http://cancercontrol.cancer.gov/brp/tcrb/monographs/19/m19_9.pdf (accessed on 2013)

An Analysis of Beijing HFMD Patients Mobility Pattern during Seeking Treatment

Zhaonan Zhu, Zhidong Cao, and Daniel Dajun Zeng

The State Key Lab of Intelligent Control and Management of Complex Systems
Institute of Automation, Chinese Academy of Sciences, Beijing, China
{zhaonan.zhu,zhidong.cao,dajun.zeng}@ia.ac.cn

Abstract. Previous epidemiological researches have studied HFMD transmission pattern, but the study on the patients mobility pattern while seeking treatment is absent. In this paper, we present a statistical analysis of the spatial-temporal pattern of the Beijing HFMD patients mobility based on a complete works dataset containing over 40,000 cases in 2010. The main findings are as follows: (1) the patents incline to take their sick children to hospitals on week-days, especially on Monday; (2) the patients living far from city center are more likely to get to hospitals in the afternoon, while the patients in the downtown in the morning; (3) patients (or their parents) either select the nearby hospitals, or the Class-A hospitals in the downtown. Furthermore, we employ a gravity model to describe the spatial mobility pattern of patients. The experiment results show a good fit.

Keywords: Hand-foot-mouth disease, mobility pattern, spatial-temporal analysis, gravity model.

1   Introduction

Hand-foot-mouth disease (HFMD), caused by Coxsackie A16 virus, can transmit among 0 to 5-year-old children through close contact, tableware and human excrement. Despite the fact that the mortality of HFMD is not much high (for example, in 2010, 19 out of 45409 cases died, so that is 0.022%), this disease brings pain to sick children and their families. Additionally, the number of HFMD patients is increasing in recent years (18445 cases in 2008, 24483 in 2009 and 45409 in 2010, from Beijing CDC), and the seasonal outbreaks of HFMD make the government suffer a high cost in preventing and controlling the transmission.

Over the past years, many researchers have conducted related research ranging from molecular biology to epidemiology. Cao et al. [1] gave an empirical analysis of the 2010 Beijing HFMD epidemiological data, revealing some spatial-temporal patterns of HFMD transmission. Chen et al. [2] analyzed epidemiologic features of Taiwan HFMD epidemic.

In the city epidemic, infected people from all over the city seek medical service. Large numbers of HFMD patients from all districts to all hospitals may cause potential risk of cross-transmission, for the patients may have close contact with the others

D. Zeng et al. (Eds.): ICSH 2013, LNCS 8040, pp. 24–30, 2013.

in the crowded public places such as buses, subway stations and hospitals. And for hospitals and public health department, the macro spatial-temporal law of the patients' mobility is very important for epidemiological survey and epidemic controlling.

Previous study mainly focused on the epidemiology mechanism, but few work studied the patients' mobility pattern when they are seeking treatment. Some human mobility-related work [4] proposed some basic spatial-temporal analysis method applied in the field of commuting data analysis, social media[5] and infectious disease[3].

The remainder of this paper is structured as follows. We begin with an introduction to the data used in this study. Then we report a spatial-temporal analysis of the data. Finally, we adopt an unconstrained gravity model to fit the commuting data, and the results analysis are also shown.

2   Data

2.1   Data Format

The 2010 Beijing HFMD case dataset provided by Beijing Center for Disease Control and Prevention (Beijing CDC) consists of detailed information of all 45409 cases that occurred in 2010. The format of the data is as follows: {caseID, gender, date of birth, profession, residential address, hospital, date of onset, date and time of visiting hospital}.

2.2   Data Preprocessing

As the raw data was filled by doctors at first, some cases' information is absent or fallacious. The cases without detailed address or the addresses of which do not belong to Beijing are removed.

We use standard place database to get all the administrative district where each case lives, and locate all the 44607 valid cases with the latitude and longitude information (accurate to the street office, which is the basic residential administrative unit in China, and there are over 340 street offices in Beijing) and all the 195 hospitals on the map of Beijing. All the 44607 cases live in 312 basic administrative units.

3   Spatial-Temporal Analysis

3.1   Wheres of the Cases

We locate all the valid cases with the geographic coordinates on the map. By generating the heat map, it is easy to see the spatial features of the cases.

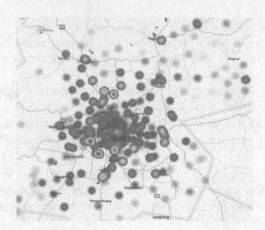

Fig. 1. The heat map of Beijing 2010 HFMD epidemic

We can see from figure 1 that the heat points are mainly located in the junction area of urban and suburban districts. It is because in those area the people commute often from suburban to urban districts. Frequent flow of people may result ín more infected cases.

3.2   Whens of Visiting Hospitals

HFMD patients are mostly 0 to 5-year-old children, so they are largely likely taken to hospitals by their adult custodians. When custodians consider when to go, they may account for both the date and the distance. We compare the different distributions of different groups of patients.

First, we compare the patients visiting hospitals on weekends and on weekdays.

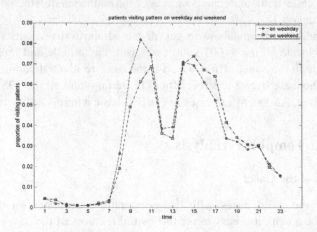

Fig. 2. The number of patients seeking treatment at different time on weekdays and weekends

Figure 2 illustrates that the patients visiting hospitals on weekdays are more willing to go in the morning, while those who seek treatment on weekends are more likely to go in the afternoon. This is because i) people tend to sleep later on weekend; ii) the doctor's duty time on weekend is shorter, and professor medicals are not always on duty on weekend, which results in less medical service seekers who long for better treatment lead by professor medicals;

Second, we compare the patients with a range of distance from living place to hospitals. We divide all the cases into 8 groups according to the distance. They are above 100 kilometers, 80-100 km, 50-80 km, 30-50 km, 15-30 km, 5-15 km, 2-5 km and below 2 km. The distributions are presented in Figure 3.

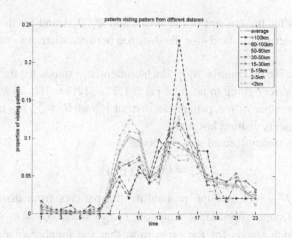

Fig. 3. The number of patients seeking treatment at different time over different distance

From the figure above we can conclude that the farther the patients are from living places to destined hospitals, the later the patient flow peaks. As the figure shows, when the distance is more than 100 kilometers, most patients come to see doctors at 15:00; however, those who are very close to hospitals (less than 2 kilometers) are most likely to visit hospitals at 10:00. This is because the patients living far from hospitals would take a long time on the way. And 10:00 and 15:00 are both the time at which doctors' workload gets the highest. This also explained why the peaks occur at 10:00 and 15:00.

4   Exploring Spatial Mobility Pattern Using Gravity Model

We consider the probability p_{ij} that a given case from area i visiting the hospital j. It is intuitive that a sick kid's parents should take some factors into consideration when they decide which hospital they would send their child to. First is the level of the hospital. A professional class-A pediatric hospital is much better than a local clinic. Second is the distance. Those too far from home are not good choice, because of the traffic cost and the time delay. These two basic factors impact parents' choice, hence patients mobility pattern.

Gravity model was first proposed by Casey in 1955[4]. It has been used to forecast trade between countries and traffic flow between provinces. It is also widely used in describing the movements of people over distance [3]. The basic idea of gravity model is to simulate the flow among two places as the gravitational force between two celestial body. The mass stands for some kind of resource that the places hold. The basic form of gravity model is:

$$p_{ij} = \alpha \frac{Q_i Q_j}{d_{ij}^2}$$

Where p_{ij} stands for the amount of the flow , and Q_i, Q_j stand for the population of district i and district j. d_{ij} stands for the distance between district i and j. And α is a scale factor.

Here we define the OD matrix $N_{i \times j}$. Each eliment n_{ij} stands for the number of patients living in district i going to hospital j (i = 1,2,...312; j = 1,2,...195). $R_i = \sum_j n_{ij}$ means the total number of the patients in district i, and $H_j = \sum_i n_{ij}$ means the total number of the patients visiting hospital j.

We consider an unconstrained gravity model:

$$p_{ij} = k Q_i^{\alpha} Q_j^{\beta} f(d_{ij})$$

Where $p_{ij} = n_{ij}/R_i$, indicates the probability the patients from district i going to hospital j. The distance impedance function $f(d_{ij}) = d_{ij}^{\gamma}$. $Q_i = n_{ij}/H_j$, and $Q_j = H_j/\sum_i \sum_j n_{ij}$, which stands for the proportion that the number of patients visiting hospital j account for of the total number (that is 44607), explains the that the hospital level is one of the factors that the parents take into consideration when they choose hospitals, because high-level hospitals always attract larger number of patients for their better medical service. The data proves this. The top 6 hospitals receive 24075 cases, and that number is over the half.

By using a standard LSM method, we get the parameters as follows. k = 5.105 × 10^{-3}, α = 0.9059, β = 0.6878, γ = −0.1997. While the R^2 = 0.6497.

After simulation with the model, the residual is found to follow a normal distribution, which indicates that the residuals of each point is independent.

The simulation result is shown below. In Figure 4, we can find that most of patients are willing to choose the hospitals which are probably about 10 kilometers away from home. And a considerable number of patients would like to go more than 10 km but less than 40 km. Those who go too far away or too near from home are not the majority. In addition, out simulation could describe such a procedure that how patients (or their parents) choose the hospitals to go while seeking treatment. Distance and the level of the hospital are the two major factors that are taken into account.

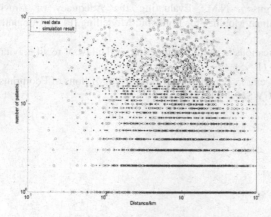

Fig. 4. The real data and the simulation result

5 Discussion

In this paper, we analyze the spatial-temporal pattern of HFMD patients seeking treatment, and an unconstrained gravity model is adopted to fit the mobility data. We find that the HFMD infected cases are mainly located in the junction area of urban and suburban districts. We also find that the temporal patterns of different group of patients seeking treatment are mostly different according to their living locations, distances to hospitals and the dates they go to see doctors. Finally, we use an unconstrained gravity model fit the mobility data. The coefficient of determination ($R^2 = 0.6497$) was not very satisfactory, it is partly because the granularity of the address information in the raw data is not fine. Over 40,000 cases located over Beijing are grouped into only 312 geographic unit, which may result in the general performance of the model.

Acknowledgments. This work is partially funded through NNSFC Grants #71025001, #71103180, #91124001, and #91024030, MOH Grants #2013ZX10004218 and #2012ZX10004801.

References

1. Cao, Z., Zeng, D., Wang, Q., Zheng, X., Wang, F.: An epidemiological analysis of the Beijing 2008 Hand-Foot-Mouth epidemic. Chinese Science Bulletin 55, 1142–1149 (2010)
2. Chen, K.T., Chang, H.L., Wang, S.T., et al.: Epidemiologic features of hand-foot-mouth disease and herpangina caused by enterovirus 71 in Taiwan, 1998-2005. Pediatrics 120, E244–E252 (2007)

3. Truscott, J., Ferguson, N.M.: Evaluating the Adequacy of Gravity Models as a Description of Human Mobility for Epidemic Modelling. PLoS Comput. Biol. 8, e1002699 (2012)
4. Casey, H.J.: Applications to traffic engineering of the law of retail gravitation. Traffic Quarterly IX(1), 23–35 (1995)
5. Cheng, Z., Caverleem, J., Lee, K., et al.: Exploring Millions of Footprints in Location Sharing Services. In: ICWSM 2011 (2011)

Phenotyping on EHR Data
Using OWL and Semantic Web Technologies

Cui Tao, Dingcheng Li, Feichen Shen, Zonghui Lian, Jyotishman Pathak,
Hongfang Liu, and Christopher G. Chute

Department of Health Sciences Research, Mayo Clinic, Rochester, MN 55905

Objective: In this paper, we introduce our efforts on using semantic web technologies to execute phenotyping algorithms on Electronic Health Records (EHR) data.

Background and Significance: In the context of our research, phenotyping refers to the algorithmic recognition of any cohort within EHR for a defined purpose. Phenotyping plays an important role on many clinical applications such as GWAS studies, clinical quality efforts, clinical decision supports, and clinical trials eligibility determination. Well-defined phenotyping algorithms span across patient diagnostics and procedure fields, laboratory values, medication use, and NLP-derived observations.

Most of the existing phenotyping algorithms usually are designed for human experts to interpret and process. They are, therefore, not directly machine executable. It is not scalable, however, to rely on manual identification of eligible patients especially with the increasing amount of EHR data adopted by healthcare systems nowadays. Automatic executions of phenotyping algorithms on EHR data are more and more desired.

Method: We propose to use semantic web and ontology-based approaches to represent phenotyping algorithms to and apply them on EHR data. The clinical elements in both phenotyping algorithms and EHR data will be represented with respect to common ontologies, so that they share the same semantics. The logics and operations in the algorithms can be represented using Web Ontology Language (OWL) Description Logic (DL), so that they can be machine-processable.

Clinical Element Model in OWL: In our approach, we use the clinical element model (CEM) [1] as the common model to represent clinical elements in both phenotyping algorithms and EHR data. CEM is an information model designed for representing clinical information in EHR systems across organizations. CEM has been adopted in the Strategic Health IT Advanced Research Project, secondary use of EHR (SHARPn) [2] as the common unified information model for unambiguous data representation, interpretation, and exchange within and across heterogeneous sources and applications. We have represented the CEM specification using the OWL. The CEM-OWL [3] representation connects the CEM content with the Semantic Web environment, which provides authoring, reasoning, and querying tools.

EHR Data in RDF: The SHARPn project provides open source tools to normalize the EHR data using common detailed clinical models (CEM) and Consolidated Health

D. Zeng et al. (Eds.): ICSH 2013, LNCS 8040, pp. 31–32, 2013.
© Springer-Verlag Berlin Heidelberg 2013

Informatics standard terminologies. Based on the CEM-OWL specification, we have implemented a framework to automatically convert the SHARPn normalized data to Resource Description Framework (RDF) format, which is a standard way to represent and exchange data in the semantic web community.

Phenotyping Algorithm in OWL DL: To investigate using OWL DL to represent the phenotyping algorithms, we use the National Quality Forum (NQF) [4] performance measures as a use case. NQF hosts hundreds of quality measure criteria. These criteria are currently represented in XML or HTML, which are not directly executable. We have summarized the operations and functions involved in the NQF measures in several categories: logic (and/or), comparison (>, < =), time, math, negation, count, order, and value set operations. We implemented a framework that can automatically parse the logics and operations from the NQF measures [5] and represent these operations using OWL DL axioms combined with Java operations.

Evaluation and Result: We evaluated the approach using three randomly selected NQF measures: NQF0001, NQF0002 and NQF0056. These three measures were run on top of a simulated RDF triple store. There are totally 390 patients in the sample data. For each patient, we have stored demographic information, laboratory records, medication history, diagnosis, encounters, and symptom descriptions. For each measure, patients eligible for the criteria are pre-determined as a gold standard for validating our reasoning results. We then applied the DL rules for each measure on top of this patient cohort. The automatic classified patient cohort was then compared with the gold standard data set to validate our approach. The evaluation result indicates that our framework can successfully represent the measure criteria faithfully and retrieve patient data correctly.

References

[1] GE/Intermountain Clinical Element Model Search,
    http://intermountainhealthcare.org/CEM/
[2] Rea, S., et al.: Building a robust, scalable and standards-driven infrastructure for secondary use of EHR data: The SHARPn project. J. Biomed. Inform. 45, 763–771 (2012)
[3] Tao, C., et al.: A semantic-web oriented representation of the clinical element model for secondary use of electronic health records data. J. Am. Med. Inform. Assoc. (December 25, 2012)
[4] Kallem, C.: Transforming clinical quality measures for EHR use. NQF refines emeasures for use in EHRs and meaningful use program. J. AHIMA 82, 52–53 (2011)
[5] Li, D., et al.: Modeling and executing electronic health records driven phenotyping algorithms using the NQF Quality Data Model and JBoss(R) Drools Engine. In: AMIA Annu. Symp. Proc., vol. 2012, pp. 532–541 (2012)

Spatial, Temporal, and Space-Time Clusters of Hemorrhagic Fever with Renal Syndrome in Beijing, China[*]

Xiangfeng Dou[1,**], Yi Jiang[2,**], Changying Lin[1,**], Lili Tian[1], Xiaoli Wang[1], Kaikun Qian[1], Xiuchun Zhang[1], Xinyu Li[1], Yanning Lyu[1], Yulan Sun[1], Zengzhi Guan[1], Shuang Li[1], and Quanyi Wang[1,**,***]

[1] Institute for Infectious Disease and Endemic Disease Control,
Beijing Center for Disease Prevention and Control, Beijing, 100013, China
bjcdcxm@126.com
[2] National Institute of Communicable Disease Control & Prevention,
Chinese Center of Disease Control & Prevention, Beijing 102206, China

Abstract. As only few cases each year, the distribution of hemorrhagic fever with renal syndrome (HFRS) had thought to be sporadic using the traditional statistical method. The cases reported between 2007 and 2012 through notifiable disease system were analyzed using SaTScan software. The spatial, temporal and space-time distribution of HFRS cases and clusters of high risk at township level was explored. The clusters in northern remote suburb, south of central urban and northern urban fringe were identified. When clusters were found, we could find evidence of risk factors easily and provide proper prevention methods ultimately. The cluster methods may have wider applications in the diseases with few cases.

Keywords: Hemorrhagic Fever with Renal Syndrome, Spatio-Temporal Analysis, Space-Time Clustering.

1 Introduction

Hemorrhagic fever with renal syndrome (HFRS) caused by Hantavirus remains an important public health problem in China[1,2,3]. As a notifiable disease, the case diagnosed clinically or confirmed by laboratory should be reported. With the greatest incidence of human disease, the annual number of reported HFRS cases in China peaked at 115804 in 1986[1]. Twenty thousand to seventy thousand HFRS cases were reported annually in 1990s[3]; the number of cases has been decreasing since then.

---

[*] This study was supported by National Key Program for Infectious Disease of China (2012ZX10004215-003-001) and Beijing Natural Science Foundation (Project No. 7133234).
[**] These authors contributed equally to this work.
[***] Corresponding author.

D. Zeng et al. (Eds.): ICSH 2013, LNCS 8040, pp. 33–40, 2013.

There were 8745 cases reported in 2009 which was the lowest number of cases in the past two decades[2]. The annual fatality rate changed from 1.00% to 2.00% in recent twenty years, with a slight increase in recently years[2].

In Beijing, after first case of HFRS was reported in 1986, only few cases were diagnosed until 1996. The number of cases reached the peak of 214 cases in 2002. Since then, cases have been decreasing in number. (Surveillance data and reports from Beijing CDC). Only 12-25 cases were reported each year in Beijing from 2007 to 2012. The cases of HFRS reported were mostly confirmed by laboratory tests and were characterized by severe bleeding diathesis and renal failure.

Focusing efforts to endemic and high-risk areas could serve as an initial, cost-effective solution[4]. As only few cases every year in Beijing, the distribution seemed to be sporadic. But the distribution of HFRS should be regular in space, time and space-time because the occurrence is determined by the distribution of their host-reservoirs[5]. So we investigated the spatial and temporal distribution of HFRS in Beijing during 2007-2012. Our aim was to characterize geographic distribution of HFRS and to identify high-risk clustering areas using space-time scan statistics.

2   Methods

2.1   Study Area

Beijing is located at the northern tip of the North China Plain, near the meeting point of Taihang mountain ranges and Yanshan mountain ranges. The terrain is roughly 38% flat and 62% mountainous. The city's climate is a rather dry, monsoon-influenced humid continental climate, characterized by hot and humid summers and generally cold, windy, and dry winters. It covers a total area of 16,807.8 km^2, divided into 14 administrative districts and 2 countries, which are subdivided into 322 townships or towns.

2.2   Data Collection

As HFRS is a notifiable disease in Beijing, China, the cases diagnosed clinically or confirmed by laboratory were reported through China Information System for Diseases Control and Prevention. Each case was investigated by the clinician through a simple structured questionnaire. The socioeconomic status such as age, sex, occupation education level, and residential address, the information on disease onset such as date of onset were collected. The computerized data sets including the above information were obtained from the Information System. The populations in each township or town were acquired from the Bureau of Statistics of Beijing. The coordinates for each township or town were also acquired from Beijing Institute of Surveying and Mapping.

2.3   The Space-Time Scan Statistic

SaTScan software (version 9.1.1) was employed [6]. The discrete Poisson model was used to retrospective space-time analysis scanning for clusters with high rates. For cluster specification in space-time analyses, the maximum spatial cluster size was limited to 5 percent of population at risk. The maximum temporal cluster size was defined as 2 months, which equals the longest incubation period of HFRS. The window Shape was circular, the number of replications was set to 999 and the significance level was set as 0.05. Case files were generated using daily aggregated numbers of HFRS cases for each township or town. Population and coordinates data were also used as inputs in SaTScan. Arcmap 9.3 was used to display space-time clusters.

3   Results

3.1   HFRS Epidemics

There were a total 107 HFRS cases reported in Beijing from 2007 to 2012, with 88 males and 19 females. The age ranged between 16 and 71 with average 38.3 year-old. There were 12-25 cases were reported each year. Compared with whole nation, the morbidity was much lower in Beijing (Table 1). Combined the data of all 6 years, the seasonal trend is easily recognized. The spring peak in May was apparent (Fig. 1).

3.2   Clustering and Cluster Detection

3.2.1   Purely Temporal Analysis
According to 2 months maximum temporal cluster size, the purely spatial analysis showed that the cases of HFRS peaked between April and June. The overall RR within the mostly likely cluster was 4.18 (P=0.012), with an observed number of cases of 11 compared with 2.87 calculated expected cases (Table 2).

3.2.2   Purely Spatial Analysis
Combined the 6 years from 2007 to 2012 as one period, 5 percent of population at risk as the maximum spatial cluster size, the purely spatial analysis showed HFRS was not distributed randomly in space (Table 3, Fig. 2). The mostly likely cluster located at remote northern suburb of Beijing, including 14 townships, where the population density was lower, plants and animals are abundant. The overall RR within the mostly likely cluster was 11.75 (P=0.000). The first secondary likely cluster located at central urban with more densely population, and the overall RR was 6.51 (P=0.029). The second likely cluster located at the north-eastern edge of urban, mainly in Chaoyang district (Fig. 2), but no significance was found (P=0.132).

3.2.3 Space-Time Analysis

The cluster both in space and time were found through the space-time analysis (Table 4, Fig. 2). The mostly likely statistically significant cluster for high incidence of HFRS was found partly overlapping with the mostly likely cluster area in purely spatial analysis, just in northern suburb in May and June, 2007. The RR within the mostly likely cluster was 70.95 (P=0.019). The secondary clusters were found no significance at 0.05 levels. But the first secondary clusters also located at central urban area, almost overlapping with the first secondary cluster area in purely spatial analysis. The second located at the north-western edge of urban, mainly in Haidian district (Fig. 2).

Table 1. Annual number of HFRS cases and death in Beijing and China between 2007 and 2012

Year	No. of cases	Beijing[*]		China[#]	
		morbidity (/100,000)	Fatality (%)	morbidity (/100,000)	Fatality (%)
2007	25	0.16	4.0	0.84	1.31
2008	17	0.11	0	0.68	1.14
2009	12	0.08	0	0.66	1.19
2010	15	0.10	0	0.71	1.24
2011	20	0.10	0	0.80	1.10
2012	18	0.09	0	-	0.73

[*] Source : China information system for diseases control and prevention ; # Source : Annual surveillance report from China CDC.

Table 2. Purely temporal analysis of HFRS in Beijing between 2007 and 2012

Year	Month	No. Obs.	No. Exp.	LLR	RR	P
2011	4.1-5.31	11	2.87	6.99	4.18	0.012
2012	5.1-5.31	6	1.34	4.46	4.73	0.108
2008	5.1-6.30	7	2.36	3.11	3.15	0.400
2007	5.1-6.30	7	2.50	2.83	2.96	0.435

No. Obs, number of observed cases; No. Exp, Number of expected cases; LLR, Log-likelihood ratio; RR, relative risk.

Table 3. Purely spatial analysis of HFRS in Beijing between 2007 and 2012

Cluster area		No. Obs.	No. Exp.	LLR	RR	P
Center	Radius (km)					
40.699288 N, 116.347014 E	33.36	8	0.73	12.12	11.75	0.000
39.865177 N, 116.394345 E	1.89	8	1.32	7.96	6.51	0.029
40.021423 N, 116.497133 E	3.39	5	0.59	6.42	9.00	0.132

No. Obs, number of observed cases; No. Exp, Number of expected cases; LLR, Log-likelihood ratio; RR, relative risk.

Table 4. Space-time analysis of HFRS in Beijing between 2007 and 2012

Cluster space		Time	No. Obs.	No. Exp.	LLR	RR	P
Center	Radius (km)						
40.416427N, 116.214590E	21.38km	2007/5/1- /6/30	4	0.059	13.03	70.95	0.019
39.879986N, 116.386027E	1.79km	2010/12/1- 2011/1/31	3	0.04	10.04	77.38	0.208
39.989944N, 116.265436E	5.21km	2012/5/1- /5/31	3	0.071	8.35	43.57	0.466

No. Obs, number of observed cases; No. Exp, Number of expected cases; LLR, Log-likelihood ratio; RR, relative risk.

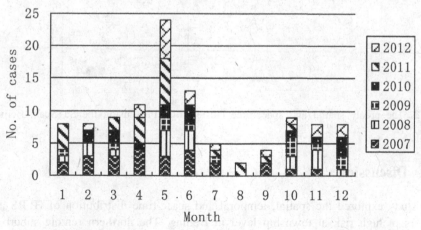

Fig. 1. Monthly number of HFRS cases in Beijing between 2007 and 2012

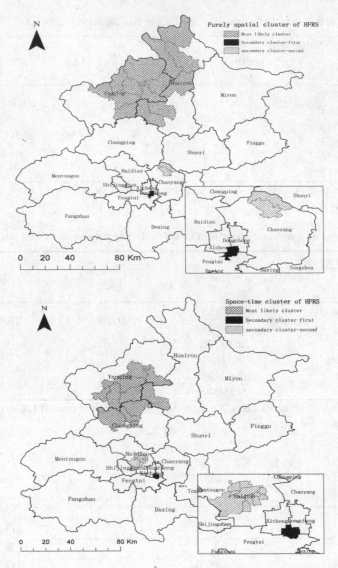

Fig. 2. The purely spatial and space-time clusters of HFRS using the SaTScan, Beijing, 2007-2012

4   Discussion

This study explored the spatial, temporal and space-time distribution of HFRS and clusters of high risk at township level in Beijing. The northern remote suburb of Beijing was constantly identified as the mostly likely cluster in both purely spatial analysis and space-time analysis. And the south of central urban area and northern urban fringe was also identified as the cluster areas. The temporal distribution peaked between April and June.

The presence of rodents and their excreta, in and around homes significantly increases the risk for human Hantavirus infection[4]. In Beijing, *Rattus norvegicus*, the most common predominant animal hosts of Seoul virus[7] were settled in areas where humans lived. Seoul virus was responsible for almost all cases of HFRS in Beijing[8,9]. In the suburb, except the influence of landscape elements[10], the residential buildings in the villages easily burrowed, the old habit reserving food supplies, agricultural activities[2] gave the local residents more chances to access *Rattus norvegicus* and their excreta. The higher risk in the south of central urban perhaps related with the history of the city. In the past, the southern urban area was the poor people zone. The preserved old houses give the *Rattus norvegicus* combatable living condition. The northern fringe of urban used to be suburb with villages in agricultural fields and wild environments. Along with the urbanization process, the urban villages, densely immigrant laborers and dirty environments became the risks of acquiring HFRS.

The spring peak in temporal distribution was decided by the host-reservoirs and pathogen in Beijing. *Apodemus agrarius* and *Rattus norvegicus* were still the most common and leading animal hosts in China[1,3]. The peak season of HFRS transmitted by *Rattus norvegicus* was spring, and it was autumn-winter transmitted by *Apodemus agrarius*[1,2,3].

The space-time scan statistic should prove useful as a tool for identifying cluster alarms that are not likely to be of public health importance[11]. The cases of HFRS had thought to be sporadic using the traditional statistical method. When statistically significant clusters were found, we could find evidence of risk factors and provide proper prevention methods ultimately. Additionally, the cluster methods developed in this study may have wider applications in the diseases with few cases.

References

1. Zhang, Y.Z., Zou, Y., Fu, Z.F.: Hantavirus infections in humans and animals, China. Emerg. Infect. Dis. 16, 1195–1203 (2010)
2. Huang, L.Y., Zhou, H., Yin, W.W.: The current epidemic situation and surveillance regarding hemorrhagic fever with renal syndrome in China (2010) (in Chinese); Liu, Z., Bing, X., Za, X., Zhi: 33, 685–691 (2012)
3. Wang, Q., Zhou, H., Han, Y.H.: Epidemiology and surveillance programs on hemorrhagic fever with renal syndrome in Mainland China (2005-2008) (in Chinese); Liu, Z., Bing, X., Za, X., Zhi: 31, 675–680 (2010)
4. Watson, D.C., Sargianou, M., Papa, A.: Epidemiology of Hantavirus infections in humans: A comprehensive, global overview. Crit. Rev. Microbiol. (2013)
5. Guan, P., Huang, D., He, M.: Investigating the effects of climatic variables and reservoir on the incidence of hemorrhagic fever with renal syndrome in Huludao City, China: a 17-year data analysis based on structure equation model. BMC Infect. Dis. 9, 109 (2009)
6. Song, C., Kulldorff, M.: Power evaluation of disease clustering tests. Int. J. Health Geogr. 2, 9 (2003)

7. Lin, X.D., Guo, W.P., Wang, W.: Migration of norway rats resulted in the worldwide distribution of seoul hantavirus today. J. Virol. 86, 972–981 (2012)
8. Zhang, X., Zhou, S., Wang, H.: Study on the genetic difference of SEO type Hantaviruses (in Chinese); Liu, Z., Bing, X., Za, X., Zhi: 21, 349–351 (2000)
9. Zuo, S.Q., Zhang, P.H., Jiang, J.F.: Seoul virus in patients and rodents from Beijing, China. Am. J. Trop. Med. Hyg. 78, 833–837 (2008)
10. Yan, L., Fang, L.Q., Huang, H.G.: Landscape elements and Hantaan virus-related hemorrhagic fever with renal syndrome, People's Republic of China. Emerg. Infect. Dis. 13, 1301–1306 (2007)
11. Kulldorff, M., Athas, W.F., Feurer, E.J.: Evaluating cluster alarms: a space-time scan statistic and brain cancer in Los Alamos, New Mexico. Am. J. Public Health 88, 1377–1380 (1998)

Extracting and Normalizing Temporal Expressions in Clinical Data Requests from Researchers

Tianyong Hao[1], Alex Rusanov[2], and Chunhua Weng[1]

[1] Department of Biomedical Informatics, Columbia University
[2] Department of Anesthesiology, Columbia University
{th2510,ar2765,cw2384}@columbia.edu

Abstract. Automatic translation of clinical researcher data requests to executable database queries is instrumental to an effective interface between clinical researchers and "Big Clinical Data". A necessary step towards this goal is to parse ample temporal expressions in free-text researcher requests. This paper reports a novel algorithm called TEXer. It uses heuristic rule and pattern learning for extracting and normalizing temporal expressions in researcher requests. Based on 400 real clinical queries with human annotations, we compared our method with four baseline methods. TEXer achieved a precision of 0.945 and a recall of 0.858, outperforming all the baseline methods. We conclude that TEXer is an effective method for temporal expression extraction from free-text clinical data requests.

Keywords: temporal expression extraction, clinical request, pattern learning.

1 Introduction

The burgeoning adoption of electronic health record (EHR) offers new opportunities to accelerate clinical and translational science (CTSA) with less expense, larger scale, and greater efficiency using the electronic data in Electronic Health Records (EHRs). Due to the enormous amount of data [1] and their complex representations, researchers interested in this data usually need to submit free-text data queries to database query specialists, who then work with the researchers to translate the requests into executable database queries. This process is labor-intensive, time-consuming, and expensive [2]. It is imperative to provide clinical researchers, who are usually not familiar with clinical databases, with an effective interface to assist in the interrogation the "Big Clinical Data" autonomously. Automatic data requests processing and query formulation methods are desired to significantly improve this process [1].

One of the major barriers to automated query formulation from clinical data requests is the recognition and extraction of temporal expressions, such as "Number of unique patient episodes from 1/1/07 - 12/31/08", contained within them. Our analysis of 400 real queries submitted to the Columbia University Medical Center (CUMC)'s Clinical Data Warehouse (CDW) by researchers revealed that over 64% of queries contain temporal expressions.

D. Zeng et al. (Eds.): ICSH 2013, LNCS 8040, pp. 41–51, 2013.

Temporal annotation of documents is crucial to a wide range of Natural Language Processing (NLP) applications, e.g., text summarization and question answering, due to its key role in chronological ordering of events [3, 4]. In response to this need, TempEval, an open evaluation challenge in the area of temporal annotation, was held in 2007 [4], 2010 [5], and 2013, and resulted in a number of systems that have experienced wide adoption. One example is HeidelTime [3], which achieved the best performance in Task A for English of the TempEval 2 challenge. In the standardization of temporal annotation schema, TimeML is a robust specification language for events and temporal expressions in text [6]. It is designed to address four problems in event and temporal expression markup: 1) Time stamping of events; 2) Ordering events with respect to one another; 3) Reasoning with contextually underspecified temporal expressions; 4) Reasoning about the persistence of events. TempEval challenge also provided detailed guidelines for Temporal Expression Annotation for English, e.g., TempEval 2010 including: 1) Noun (including Proper Nouns): e.g., *today*; 2) Noun Phrase: e.g., *Friday night*; 3) Adjective: e.g., *current*; 4) Adverb: e.g. *recently*; 5) Adjective or Adverb Phrase: e.g. *half an hour long*.

For temporal extraction methods, TempEx aims at TIMEX2 standard for recognizing normalized time expressions. TempEx handles both absolute times (e.g., *June 2, 2003*) and relative times (e.g., *Thursday*) by means of a number of tests on the local context. GUTime extends the capabilities of the TempEx. Lexical triggers like *yesterday* as well as words which indicate a positional offset (e.g., *next month*) are resolved based on computing direction with respect to a reference time. More advanced temporal extraction methods were developed since 2010. For example, Heideltime win best system for the extraction and normalization of English temporal expressions in TempEval-2 challenge. However, all these systems are conducted primarily on newspaper and narrative texts and did not work well on clinical texts.

Among most recent research on temporal annotation from clinical texts, Sohn et al. proposed a comprehensive temporal information detection method from clinical text [7]. Tang et al. presented a hybrid system for temporal information extraction from clinical text [8]. Tao et al. proposed Ontology-based time information representation of vaccine adverse events in VAERS for temporal analysis [9]. Li & Patrick introduced a method to extract temporal information from electronic patient records [10]. Galescu & Blaylock built a corpus of clinical narratives annotated with temporal information [11]. Luo et al. used Conditional Random Fields for Extracting Temporal Constraints from Clinical Research Eligibility Criteria [12]. However, it is difficult to evaluate their performances without open-available systems. In addition, most of these systems process narrative clinical texts rather than user-generated high complexity texts.

The narrative texts are different from the free text requests authored by clinical researchers. The presence of a large amount of International Classification of Diseases (ICD), Admit Discharge Transfer (ADT), Current Procedural Terminology (CPT) codes, age related information, and biomedical abbreviations dramatically increase the complexity of this type of text. In addition, the variety of representations particularly uncommon temporal expression formats, e.g., "March 20=06", as well as noise data (spelling mistakes) made the text difficult to process. As a result, we tested a variety of public tools for temporal information extraction but none worked satisfactorily for clinical research authored queries.

Therefore, we developed a novel automated method - Temporal Expression Extractor (TEXer), for clinical request formulation. TEXer combines heuristic rule and pattern learning to identify temporal expressions in data requests authored by researchers. Patterns, as the representations of multi-temporal expressions, are learned from annotated training datasets and calculated with confidence values by matching with all training texts. When applying on testing data, the validated patterns are used to judge candidate temporal expressions extracted using heuristic rules. The identified temporal expressions are further normalized according to TimeML standard.

Our experiments used 400 real queries submitted to CUMC's CDW. These queries were manually annotated and validated by two independent raters, a clinical researchers and a computer scientist. 100 queries were used as training data and the other 300 were used as the gold standard for the testing data. We used Heideltime, GUTime, IllinoisTemporalExtractor, and NLTK TimeX module as baselines for comparison.

2   Methods

Our approach called TEXer combines heuristic rule and pattern learning methods for temporal expression identification. TEXer initially utilizes a group of heuristic rules representing the features of observed temporal expressions from a training dataset to capture temporal expression candidates. After that, a group of text patterns are extracted automatically based on the sentences containing annotated temporal expressions in training dataset. The trained patterns are then matched with all sentences to calculate pattern confidence. The validated patterns are ranked and applied on new texts for judging candidates that not able to be decided by solely heuristic rules. The extracted temporal expressions are finally normalized following TimeML, a well-adopted markup language. The framework of the approach is shown as Figure 1.

Each temporal expression is represented as a three-tuple $te_i = <t_i, a_i, v_i>$, where t_i is the expression itself as it occurs in the textual document, a_i represents the type attribute of the expression, and v_i is the normalized value. We used four temporal types, namely *Date*, *Time*, *Duration*, and *Set*, following TimeML standard. The normalized value represents the temporal semantics of an expression as it is specified by TimeML, regardless of the expression used in the document. The goal of TEXer is to extract the temporal expression t_i and to correctly assign the type attributes a_i and normalize the expression into date value v_i, respectively.

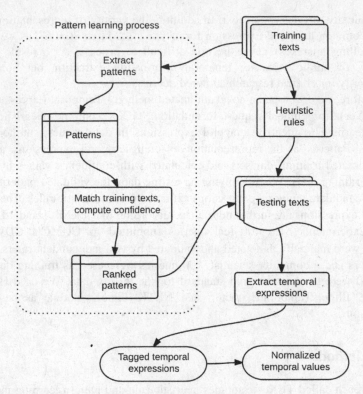

Fig. 1. The framework of TEXer using heuristic rules and pattern learning methods

We use TimeX3 as the annotation of temporal expressions following the standard temporal expression schema - TimeML. Temporal expressions are in XML format, e.g., <TIMEX3 tid="t1" type="Duration" value="P2M">2 months</TIMEX3>. Each TIMEX3 is assigned one of the following types: Date, Time, Duration, and Set. The format of the value attribute is determined by the type of TIMEX3. For instance, a Duration has a value that begins with the letter 'P' since durations represent a period of time. This will be elaborated on below in the value section. In addition, some optional attributes are used for specific types of temporal expressions.

Based on annotated temporal texts, we extract temporal expressions and observe a group of representation features. These features are further categorized and summarized as a list of heuristic rules for identifying temporal expression candidates. As an example of the rule generation procedure, 137 temporal expressions from 100 manually annotated queries (Table 1) were manually categorized into features. Features, which represent the formats of these expressions, are assigned based on the context of the temporal expression in the original context. The features are then converted into heuristic rules. Note that these rules contain not only regular expressions, but also matching rules, e.g., filter age information. The extracted expressions and their features and heuristic rules are presented in Table 2.

Table 1. Examples of temporal expressions contained in 100 manually annotated queries

present; 1/2001; 72 hours; 6 MONTHS; January 1st, 2003; 6 MONTHS; January 1st, 2006; 1/1/99; January, 2004; January 1, 2001; 14 days; 90 DAYS; last year; June, 2004; 5/31/2005; December 2005; 9/18/2003; 9/11/62; 90 days; January, 2005; year 2; May 1, 2006; March 20; 72 hours; 1/1/1996; 2 years; January 1, 1997; 72 hours; 2006; 12 months; current; 1995; 1/23/98; first year; 14 days; 2000; Nov 1 2005; 2000; 14 days; 2005; november of 2003;

Table 2. Examples of observed features and generated heuristic rules

Expressions	Features	Heuristic rules
December 1-7, 2003	[SLOT=month]<S= >[SLOT=day] <S=->[SLOT=day]<S=,><S=> [SLOT=year]	*(?<!(\w|\d|<|>|/))('+[month]+r' \d{1,2}(- |-| -|-)\d{1,2}(, |,|)\d{2,4})(?!(\w|\d|<|>|/))*
May 1, 2006	[SLOT=month]<S= >[SLOT=day] <S=,><S=> [SLOT=year]	*(?<!(\w|\d|<|>|/))('+[month]+r'(- |-| -|- |)\d{1,2}(, |,|)\d{1,4})(?!(\w|\d|<|>|/))*
January 1st, 2006	[SLOT=month]<S= >[SLOT=day] (LIST=st, nd, rd, th)<S=,><S=> [SLOT=year]	*(?<!(\w|\d|<|>|/))('+[month]+'(- |-| -|- |)\d{1,2}(st|nd|rd|th)(, |,|)\d{1,4})(?!(\w|\d|<|>|/))*
Aged 20 years old	Negative feature	*Filter if char distance(feature, [age|ages|aged|aging]) < n*

Certain temporal expressions are contextually connected to each other in the original text, e.g., "from Jan 2011 to Dec 2011". There is potential for using these contextual relationships to define patterns for temporal information extraction. However, blind application of such patterns may lead to incorrect extraction of non-temporal information, e.g., falsely extracting ICD9 codes as dates in the example "from 070.22 to 070.44". Therefore, an algorithm capable of automated pattern learning and validation is preferred.

We propose a pattern learning algorithm based on a manually annotated original text. The core idea is to mine all the patterns that contain single or multiple temporal expressions and then match each pattern with all its occurrences within the original annotated text to calculate its confidence. The confidence is defined as the percentage of correct matching with temporal expressions over all matching. The patterns are evaluated in terms of possible correct matching and miss-match, and therefore achieve more reliable results. The algorithm consists of six steps: 1) replace original annotation tags and temporal expressions with a specific tag; 2) extract temporal combinations by mining patterns containing the specific tag as candidate patterns; 3) extract atomic pattern by mining context containing the specific tags as candidate patterns; 4) combine all candidate patterns and calculate their frequency; 5) match each candidate pattern with original text to calculate its confidence value; 6) filter candidate patterns by confidence value to get final patterns.

For example, a sentence "PED for acute asthma exacerbation from <TI>1/2004</TI> to <TI>1/2005</TI> stratified by age", where "<TI></TI>" is a temporal annotation tag generated automatically. After that, our algorithm replaces the annotations with tags as "PED for acute asthma exacerbation from <TE> to <TE> stratified by age". Based on this, a group of candidate patterns are extracted (Table 3).

Table 3. Examples of learned patterns from traning dataset before confidence filtering

Exacerbation from <TE> to <TE> stratified
Exacerbation from <TE> to <TE>
from <TE> to <TE> stratified
from <TE> to <TE>
<TE> to <TE> stratified
<TE> to <TE>

Next, all the frequency values of candidate patterns are calculated and matched with all occurrences of the pattern in the full original text to calculate confidences. For example, "<TE> to <TE>" is matched with "from <TI>January 1995</TI> to <TI>present</TI>" and "drawn from patients admitted to 9 Garden North Milstein". Since the first match successfully tags a temporal expression, its confidence is calculated as 0.5. Only pattern candidates with confidences larger than a threshold are considered as validated patterns to be used in temporal information extraction. We empirically set confidence threshold here as 0.7, which can be generalized by a systematic comparison of precision and recall on a training dataset. Eventually, the extracted temporal expressions are classified into types and normalized into values by a normalization function inside TEXer. For example, "to current day" is annotated as "to <TIMEX3 tid="t1" Type="Date" Value="2013-05-13">current day</TIMEX3>", where "DATE" is a type attribute and "2013-05-13" is the normalized value corresponding to a reference date.

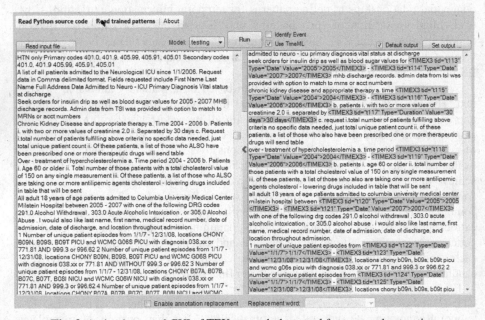

Fig. 2. An implemented GUI of TEXer as a desktop tool for temporal extraction

TEXer is available in a variety of user interfaces, Graphical User Interface (GUI), web-based, and command line, and is easily adaptable to different user needs. In addition to normal TimeX3 format processing, it can also output other types of annotations, e.g., user-defined short tags for fast comparison purposes. The annotations can be visualized by different colors, e.g., *Temporal* as green color and *Event* as blue. Figure 2 illustrates the GUI of TEXer as an example.

3   Evaluation

3.1   Baselines

We use four public, state-of-the-art, temporal expression processing systems mainly designed for news or narrative texts as baseline methods.

1. Heideltime[1]

HeidelTime is a multilingual temporal tagger that extracts temporal expressions from documents and normalizes them according to the TIMEX3 annotation standard, which is part of TimeML [3]. HeidelTime is a rule-based system and uses different normalization strategies depending on the domain of the documents that are to be processed. HeidelTime was the best system for the extraction and normalization of English temporal expressions from documents in the TempEval-2 challenge in 2010. It uses a group of precision-optimized rule sets in assigning the value attributes (85% values are assigned correctly). In addition, the type attribute was correctly assigned to 96% of the extracted expressions.

2. GUTime - The Tarsqi Toolkit[2]

GUTime extends TempEx to handle time expressions based on the TimeML TIMEX3 standard, which allows a functional style of encoding offsets in time expressions [13]. For example, *last week* could be represented not only by the time value but also by an expression that could be evaluated to compute the value, namely, that it is *the week* preceding the week of the document date. GUTime also handles a variety of ACE TIMEX2 expressions not covered by TempEx, including durations, a variety of temporal modifiers, and European date formats. GUTime has been benchmarked on training data from the Time Expression Recognition and Normalization task at 0.85, 0.78, and 0.82 of F-measure for timex2, text, and val fields, respectively.

3. IllinoisTemporalExtractor[3]

The Illinois Temporal Extractor processes documents and extracts temporal expressions, relating them to each other and optionally to a reference date [14]. The Temporal Extractor is intended to be used programmatically. Some rudimentary

---

[1] https://code.google.com/p/heideltime/
[2] http://www.timeml.org/site/tarsqi/modules/gutime/index.html
[3] http://cogcomp.cs.illinois.edu/page/software_view/
  IllinoisTemporalExtractor

command-line functionality is provided principally to allow users to test that it is working properly. The Extractor works only for English plain text. It also provided an online version.

4. NLTK Contrib library[4]

\NLTK Contrib repository, containing a module called timex.py that can tag temporal expressions, is an open source library widely used for NLP [15]. Certain ambiguous temporal expressions, e.g., "this week", or "next month", are relative to a specific reference time (e.g., the text was written). The Timex module provides a way to annotate text so these expressions can be extracted for further analysis.

3.2   Datasets

We used 400 real free-text queries submitted to via an on-line submission system for the Columbia University Medical Center Clinical Data Warehouse. Two annotators, a clinical researcher and a computer scientist, manually tagged all temporal expressions from randomly selected 400 queries. The overlap between the annotators was calculated as 87.4%. Disagreements were classified as minor, partial, and distinct. Most cases were minor (e.g., "the <TI>past year</TI>" versus "<TI>the past year</TI>") and partial (e.g. "through <TI>March 20=06</TI>" versus "through <TI>March 20</TI>=06") disagreements and were resolved by following TimeML annotation guideline. The 1 case of distinct disagreement "- <TI>date query is run</TI>" versus "- date query is run" was resolved by considering it a temporal expression after a discussion between the two annotators. Of the 400 annotated queries 100 were used as the Training dataset and remaining 300 queries as the Testing dataset.

The 400 queries contained a total of 1,044 sentences (2.61 sentences per query). 2,397 tokens were extracted indicating the sentences are short. A total of 553 temporal expressions were annotated (1.38 expressions per query). Note that even though TEXer contains an *Event* extraction function, our evaluation focused only on temporal expression extraction rather than *Event* or *Relation* extraction because some temporal expressions are associated with patients' records rather than certain events. A detailed summary of the dataset is presented in Table 4.

Table 4. Summary of traning and testing datasets

Dataset	#Queries	#Sentences	#Tokens	#Temporal expressions	Average #ex./query
Training dataset	100	257	694	155	1.55
Testing dataset	300	787	1,703	398	1.33
Total	400	1,044	2,397	553	1.38

---

[4] https://github.com/nltkThe

3.3   Results

Using the training dataset, TEXer created 21 heuristic rules and learned 65 patterns for temporal expression extraction. Table 5 shows patterns and examples categorized into Date, Time, Duration, and Set types.

Table 5. Learned patterns and exammples categorized into four types

Type	Learned patterns	Examples
Date	discharged in <TI>	*surgery patients discharged in 2005*
	outcomes BEGINNING <TI>	*cardiovascular outcomes BEGINNING 6 MONTHS*
Time	within <TI> of admission	*within 72 hours of admission to the hospital*
	with <TI> prior to	*starting with 72 hours prior to the mid-date of the patients admission*
Duration	admitted between <TI> and <TI>	*admitted between January and June, 2004*
	study period <TI> - <TI>	*study period January 1st, 2003 - January 1st, 2006*
Set	issued on a <TI> basis	*issued on a monthly basis*
	Periodically <TI>	*data sent to a central dataset periodically perhaps monthly*

After training TEXer we applied it as well as the four baselines methods to the same testing dataset. The results are shown as Table 6. Heideltime achieved a precision of 0.828, and a recall of 0.822, the best in the four baseline methods. NLTK Timex performed the worst with a precision of 0.255 and recall of 0.223. Our TEXer performed the best of all tested systems, achieving the highest scores for precision, recall and F1-score.

Table 6. Preformance comparsion of Texer and four baseline methods

Methods	#Temporal	#Correct	Precision	Recall	F1 Score
TEXer	360	340	**0.945**	**0.858**	**0.899**
Heideltime	395	327	0.828	0.822	0.825
IllinoisTemporalExtractor	352	287	0.814	0.721	0.765
GUTime	101	88	0.871	0.221	0.353
NLTK Timex	106	27	0.255	0.223	0.238

4   Discussions

4.1   Errors Due to Dataset Complexity

By analyzing annotation errors from TEXer and the four baseline methods, we found certain errors were caused by unique features of clinical data requests, which contain a large amount of ICD9, ADT, CPT codes (e.g., 147 ICD9 code instances found in 100 randomly selected queries) which are numerical codes for example, "ER 6/1/06 - 12/31/06, specifically Direct Admissions 32467 Out - Inpatient Transfer 32472 ER Visit 48678 Discharge 32469". NLTK Timex incorrectly tagged most of these ICD9 codes as temporal expressions, severely degrading its performance. The queries also contain a large number of quantity and unit combinations, which are often identified as temporal expression by regular expression matching. For example, IllinoisTemporalExtractor identified "1000" in "1000 mg in 20 ml" cases as a temporal expression, decreasing its performance.

In addition, some user-specific temporal expressions are in special format. For example, "March 20=06", "through current day =20", "March 3/06", and "a patient started HD 1/00" are in very uncommon formats, causing both TEXer and baseline systems to only partially tag them. Lastly, noise data, such as spelling mistakes affected performance of all the methods. For example, "1992-pr!esent" and "from1995 to the present" (no space between "from" and "1995"). User generated free-text queries will always suffer from these types of errors and the development of methods that are tolerant to them are necessary. TEXer shows big improvement on this issue.

4.2   Errors Due to Methodology

Though most of the errors resulted due to the highly complexity of the dataset, some were caused by methodology. GUTime integrated in the TTK tool over relies on Part-of-Speech (POS), separating cases such as "1/1/1997" into "1/1/ <TIMEX3 tid="t3" TYPE="DATE" VAL="1997"><lex pos="CD">1997 </lex></TIMEX3>". The method also tagged "the present" as *Event* rather than temporal expression due to POS. Heideltime missed "present", "daily", and some abbreviations, e.g., "24 hrs". It also erroneously tagged special codes as temporal expressions, e.g., "2484" in "CHEM-7 Creatinine Measurement MEd code 2484". IllinoisTemporalExtractor erroneously tagged all instances of "fall" as temporal expressions even though none were deemed to be temporal by the annotator (all related to the action of falling down, not the season). It also missed "present" and minutes, e.g., "1 min". NLTK did not perform well on month abbreviation and year combinations, e.g., "Jan. 2008" (only "2008" was tagged). In addition, all baseline methods tagged age information as temporal, e.g., "all patients aged 18 years old" was tagged at "18 years". Age should be distinguished from temporal information as it is an independent and important feature. TEXer processed most of the above cases but erroneously tagged some abbreviations. For example, "MAR" in "MAR info tables" and "Jan" in "MD Jan Quaegebeur" were tagged as *Month*.

5 Conclusions

Clinical researcher-authored free text requests for EHR data pose a unique information extraction challenge. TEXer, a heuristic rule and pattern learning based, temporal extraction rule outperforms existing tools when applied to this complex dataset. This robust tool can be used to assist in the automation of query processing. We intend to continue TEXer development by improving the performance of normalization, event extraction, and link identification.

References

1. Lonsdale, D.W., Tustison, C., Parker, C.G., Embley, D.W.: Assessing Clinical Trial Eligibility with Logic Expression Queries. Data & Knowledge Engineering 66(1), 3–17 (2008)
2. Hruby, G.W., Boland, M.R., et al.: Characterization of the Biomedical Query Mediation Process. In: Proc. of AMIA 2013 Clinical Research Informatics Summit, San Francisco, CA, March 18-22, pp. 89–93 (2013)
3. Strötgen, J., Gertz, M.: Heideltime: High Quality Rule-based Extraction and Normalization of Temporal Expressions. In: Proc. of the Workshop on Semantic Evaluation, pp. 321–324. ACL (2010)
4. Pustejovsky, J., Verhagen, M.: Semeval-2010 Task 13: Evaluating Events, Time Expressions, and Temporal Relations (tempeval-2). In: Proc. of the Workshop on Semantic Evaluations, pp. 112–116. ACL (2009)
5. Verhagen, M., Sauri, R., Caselli, T., Pustejovsky, J.: Semeval-2010 Task 13: Tempeval-2. In: Proc. of the Workshop on Semantic Evaluation, pp. 57–62. ACL (2010)
6. Pustejovsky, P., Castaño, J., et al.: Timeml: Robust Specification of Event and Temporal Expressions in Text. In: Proc. of the IWCS-5 Fifth International (2003)
7. Sohn, S., Wagholikar, K., Li, D., et al.: Comprehensive Temporal Information Detection from Clinical Text: Medical Events, Time, and Tlink Identification. J. Am. Med. Inform. Assoc. (2013), doi:10.1136/amiajnl-2013-00162
8. Tang, B., Wu., Y., et al.: A Hybrid System for Temporal Information Extraction from Clinical Text. J. Am. Med. Inform. Assoc. (2013), doi:10.1136/amiajnl-2013-001635
9. Tao, C., He, Y., Poland, G., Chute, C., Yang, H.: Ontology-based Time Information Representation of Vaccine Adverse Events in Vaers for Temporal Analysis. Journal of Biomedical Semantics 3(13) (2012)
10. Li, M., Patrick, J.: Extracting Temporal Information from Electronic Patient Records. In: Proc. of AMIA Annu. Symp. Proc., pp. 542–551 (2012)
11. Galescu, L., Blaylock, N.: A Corpus of Clinical Narratives Annotated with Temporal Information. In: Proc. of International Health Informatics Symposium, pp. 715–720 (2012)
12. Luo, Z., Johnson, S., Lai, A., Weng, C.: Extracting Temporal Constraints from Clinical Research Eligibility Criteria Using Conditional Random Fields. In: Proc. of AMIA Annual Symposium, pp. 843–852 (2011)
13. Mani, I., Wilson, G.: Automating Temporal Annotation with Tarsqi. In: Proc. of 38th Annual Meeting of the ACL, pp. 69–76 (2000)
14. Zhao, R., Do, Q., Roth, D.: A Robust Shallow Temporal Reasoning System. In: Proc. of NAACL-HLT Demo. (2012)
15. Bird, S.: Nltk: the Natural Languagetoolkit. In: Proc. of the COLING/ACL 2006 Interactive Presentation Sessions, pp. 69–72 (2006)

Exploring Interoperability Approaches and Challenges in Healthcare Data Exchange

Shalini Bhartiya[1] and Deepti Mehrotra[2]

[1] IITM (GGSIPU), New Delhi, India
[2] ASCS, Noida, India
shalinibhartiya69@gmail.com, dmehrotra@amity.edu

Abstract. Today e-health data and its usage in various dimensions is one of the most discussed issues. The nature of health data is heterogeneous and distributed, accessed through varied formats and architectures supporting different vocabularies. Interoperable electronic Health Record (EHR) systems are the most important enabling tools on the road to patient-centric care, a lifeline for continuity of care and support to mobility of patients. Also, hospitals refer cases to other hospitals located in same or different cities or countries altogether leading to sharing of information. This generates the reason to study the suitability of available models and protocols enabling exchange of sensitive and time critical health information during open-ended transmission. The issue of sharing data in integrated applications is highly significant and affected by various implicit and explicit factors in terms of technologies and adoption by health providers. Varied architectural approaches are implemented by vendors for designing a HIS (Hospital Information System) without giving any consideration to integrated and interoperable sharing of data. Such disparate systems are best when used in isolation but very weak when try to talk with each other. This paper aims to review issues related creation of architectures in the perspective of sharing of electronic health records and the challenges faced by them in an interoperable environment.

Keywords: Architectures, E-Health, EHR, Exchange, HIS, Interoperability, Models.

1 Introduction

Electronic health record is the outcome of the treatments a patient receives from various care-providers during his lifetime. This manifests itself in a variety of forms ranging from a detailed general record capturing clinical detail at the primary care surgery, through specialist clinical databases for particular areas of care, to the more general patient administration record created and held at the acute and secondary care hospital. Potential users of E-Health data are stated in Figure 1.

Interoperability in general is defined as the ability of two or more systems exchange information [1-2]. Interoperability of EHR defined in ISO (ISO TC 215, ISO/TR 20514, 2005) is "the ability of two or more applications being able to

D. Zeng et al. (Eds.): ICSH 2013, LNCS 8040, pp. 52–65, 2013.
© Springer-Verlag Berlin Heidelberg 2013

communicate in an effective manner without compromising the content of transmitted EHR."

EHR interoperability enables better workflows and reduced ambiguity, and allows data transfer among EHR systems and health care stakeholders. Ultimately, it improves the delivery of health care by making the right data available at the right time to the right people. To achieve effective, efficient, coordinated care, data must be shared seamlessly between health care organizations, physicians, pharmacists, nurses, patients etc.[16] While E-health tools and services are now widespread and have been revolutionizing the healthcare sector in recent years, all too often health authorities, hospitals, or doctors have selected and implemented their own individual systems. Managing these different sub-systems has been difficult requiring dedicated gateways with respect to the number of systems to be connected.

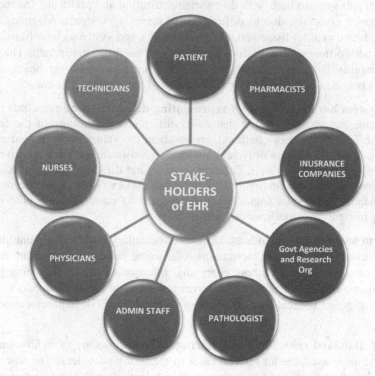

Fig. 1. Stakeholders of Electronic Health Records

Some generic models of interoperability have been proposed by researchers [3-4], which focused on semantic, syntactic, network and basic connectivity interoperability.

Semantic interoperability is most needed when electronic health record (EHR) data are to be shared and combined from different systems (or across diverse modules within a large system). Full semantic interoperability is required across heterogeneous EHR systems in order to gain the benefits of computerized support for reminders, alerts, decision support, workflow management and evidence based healthcare, i.e. to improve effectiveness and reduce clinical risks.

Integration is generally considered to go beyond mere interoperability to involve some degree of functional dependence. Interoperable systems are by necessity compatible, but the converse is not necessarily true. Apart from incurring huge cost, lack of standardization of interoperable systems, replacing legacy systems not designed to communicate and many such complex issues needs to be addressed with respect to sharing of electronic health records across organizations.

2   Challenges to Sharing of Health Data in Interoperable Environment

The functionalities of Hospital Information System (HIS) depend on higher heterogeneity of sub-systems built with different specification and protocols. Interoperability becomes a constraint due to differences in operating systems, programming language and hardware for those sub-systems. Devices and systems come from different vendors with different network interfaces but still need to interoperate. The need of interoperability is clearly visible but achieving interoperability in health data exchange is bounded with various constraints, few of them as listed below.

Every system has its own way of representing data: In this case, records referring to the same entity can represent that entity differently due to any of the following factors: different keys (key-conflicts), errors about the values of the record attributes (attribute-conflicts) and possibly schema-level inconsistencies, such as different descriptions (formats, types, etc.), different models, and different structural representations. Some of the problems with data standards and exchange arise due to the fact that standards and terminologies are not designed to serve multiple purposes thus resulting in significant inefficiencies and overhead.

One term has multiple meanings: Different vocabulary leads to different interpretation of similar terms. Two or more terms refer to the same concept but are not easily recognized as synonyms. Without contextual information the full meaning in health data remain ambiguous leading to incorrect reporting or decision-support behaviour. A single standard vocabulary is unlikely to meet all the EHR requirements of an organization.

Lack of Standard rules for Data Sharing: Who will decide as to how much data should be made available for referral cases to the health providers? The cost and benefits of data sharing should be viewed in ethical, institutional, legal, and professional dimensions. It needs to clear if data can or cannot be shared, under what circumstances, by and with whom, and for what purposes.

Lack of integration between disparate systems resulting in generation of independent silos of EHR storage: In order for interoperability within a hospital or health system, the network and infrastructure need capabilities to collect, aggregate and manage each data type. True interoperability involves intelligent bridging, not just connecting information.

Data Exchange Constraint: Due to a lack of shared infrastructure among hospital IT and EHR systems, the healthcare industry has not reached the widespread interoperability it needs to foster preventive care and effective population health management. No centralized storage of health records of every citizen and manual transfer of records from one hospital to another forfeit the dream of making the data available for efficient and timely treatment of the patient irrespective of time and place.

EHR Linkage Problem: Creation of multiple versions of EHR of the patient due to independent and non-integrated systems placed at various locations where patient visited for treatment is another major problem. Such linkage problem [15] is not only external but also is found in internal departments of the same system. Correctness and completeness of data is at stake when data cannot be recognized by a single unique identifier across the systems.

Different requirements when exchanging data: Different network requirements from different departments can also dictate changes in network design and deployment. For example, the radiology department requires significantly more bandwidth because of the high volume of image files passed between modalities such as Computed Tomography (CT), Magnetic Resonance Imaging (MRI), and Digital Radiography (DR) to the Picture Archiving and Communications System (PACS) and then to radiology viewing workstations. As more and more critical patient information migrates to the network, the network must provide adequate bandwidth, security, and data availability to ensure timely delivery of patient information to medical staff and doctors.

3 Literature Review

New metadata techniques and standards are evolving for describing semantics, but these are not fully mature nor are they widely deployed. Component-based development is a software engineering methodology, which supports the development of rich software applications by dividing them into independent components. The common selected approaches[32] that drive interoperability are OMG's Common Object Request Broker Architecture (CORBA), Microsoft DCOM/COM+ family, .NET Framework, Sun's Java 2 Enterprise Edition (J2EE), and World Wide Web Consortium's (W3C) extensible Markup Language (XML) based Web Services.

Table 1 list various architectures enabling interoperability in general, with their features and limitations. It also shows some of the approaches or models in healthcare based on the said architecture.

Table 1. Generic Architectures to Interoperability Modelled on Healthcare Systems

Architecture	Features	Limitations	Models designed for Healthcare
CORBA ver. 2 Developed in	Define interfaces between compo-	Any modification of legacy sys-	Synapses approach[17]: three-

Table 1. (*Continued*)

Architecture	Features	Limitations	Models designed for Healthcare
1994 by Object Operating Management Group(OMG)	nents, and specifies standard services such as persistent object services, directory and naming services and transaction services Relieves from many of the chores of establishing the communication formats, mapping applications to one another and maintaining the links	tems could be costly and time consuming. Defined by consensus and compromise and is not perfect This conflicts with the reality of corporate security policies [20].	year project funded under the European Union's (EU's) Fourth Framework Health Telematics Programme. Synapses has based its design around the work of CEN TC/251/PT1- 011. Synapses sets out to solve problems of sharing data between autonomous information systems by providing generic and open means to combine healthcare records or dossiers consistently, simply, comprehensibly, and securely, whether the data pass within a single healthcare institution or between institutions. Experience: Time Delays between client and server when large amount of data is transmitted CPR subsystem[18] that retrieves and stores EHRs in the object-oriented database via internet Intra-ORB Protocol (IIOP). SIGOBT archi-

Table 1. (*Continued*)

Architecture	Features	Limitations	Models designed for Healthcare
			tecture for HL7 version 2.2 with Object Request Brokers (ORB) simplifying messaging [19] The Special Interest Group on Object Brokering Technolo-gies(SIGOBT) group has been exploring how to share HL7 data in the environments of two object brokering environments i.e. Microsoft OLE and CORBA. The HL7 Version 2.X Object Mapping Specification (OMS) prescribes the process of translating given HL7 protocol
COM/DCOM Developed in 1994by Microsoft	Uses a combination of specific data to guarantee the uniqueness of each generated identifier, Global Unique Identifier (GUID). A component model supports distributed components by defining common data representations and invocation semantics Provides Basic component interop-	Requires information of the remote systems before functioning and eventually leads into modifying the legacy systems that are not complied with COM standards	PACMEDNET [24] focuses on prototyping solutions for solving interoperability problemsPresents a structured view of data collected from medical treatment facilities around the world. HOSxP[25] uses client-server architecture and implements DCOM

Table 1. (*Continued*)

Architecture	Features	Limitations	Models designed for Healthcare
	erability, Versioning, Language independence and Transparent cross-process interoperability		
.NET Framework Developed in 2000 and Java[5] based platform	Provides cross-language platform where classes and objects are interchangeable and reusable. Achieve interoperability through remote invocation or messaging.	Manipulating information within the document itself can rapidly become unwieldy. Also, there is no intrinsic way of using a parser to map objects in the XML document to classes either in Java or in .NET. Can only be implemented with the presence and requirement of Java Virtual Machine (JVM) in remote and local component of the system involved	Infosys Health Benefit Exchange Healthcare / Application Development using SharePoint / .NET CitiusTech Healthcare Software Engineering using .NET, Java/J2EE,WPF smartData Offshore Health Care application Development using .NET, ASP, AJAX JAnaemia[26] based on the EHCR architecture proposed in the ENV 13606:1999 standard, published by the CEN/TC251 committee The Brazilian National Healthcare System developed in Eclipse based on EJB 2.1 + Struts.
GUMO (General User Model Ontology)[7] and OWL (Semantic Web language)	Commonly accepted top level ontology for user and context models. This ontology is	The problem of syntactical and structural differences between existing user model-	Clinical E-Science Framework (CLEF)[27], Patient Chronicle Model (PCM)

Table 1. (*Continued*)

Architecture	Features	Limitations	Models designed for Healthcare
extension of Resource Description Framework (RDF) developed by W3c in 2004	represented in a modern semantic web language like OWL and is available for all user-adaptive systems at the same time via internet. OWL has very large vocabulary[21] with rich variety of annotations	ing and context systems could be overcome with a commonly accepted taxonomy, specialized for user modeling tasks. Computational complexity is polynomial[31]	based OOPs concepts provided by OWL ontology
Web Services[10]	XML based protocols that provides fundamental blocks for creating distributed applications Allows any piece of software to communicate with each other in a standardized XML Messaging system	Many WS-*[12] specifications are in early adoption phase, and could potentially reveal interoperability issues with different stacks.	Web Service-Based[28] Integrated Healthcare Information System (WSIHIS)
Open Systems	set of protocols, standards, and a hierarchical structure [6]from which software and hardware are built that ensure passing of information in an integrated and interoperable manner	All open source editing tools run into memory problem when dealing with very large terminologies	DHIS Open-source district health management information system and data warehouse (license: BSD license) HRHIS Open-source human resource for HIS for management of human resources for health developed by University of Dares Salaam, Department of Computer Science, for Ministry of Health and

Table 1. (*Continued*)

Architecture	Features	Limitations	Models designed for Healthcare
			Social Welfare (Tanzania) and funded by the Japan International Cooperation Agency (JICA)(license: G PLv3)
Service-Oriented Architectures	Provides a uniform means to offer, discover, interact with, and use capabilities to produce desired effects consistent with measurable preconditions and expectations. It provides a means to make services interoperable regardless of the programming language used, location, or platform of a simulation or model	Transformations become unmanageable and extensions and the complexity of writing XSLT code reduce the interoperability and portability of these transforms	CONNECT [14]: provides a SOA based "Platform for Participation" for Health Information Exchange HL7 System Design Reference Model (HER-SD RM) Built on Healthcare SOA Reference Architecture Oracle SOA Suite [29] for Health Care Integration enables advanced capabilities, which allows health care organizations to simplify and jump-start their integration initiatives with a highly flexible platform for collaboration across all health care domains
ISO/EN 13606 Part 1[4], openEHR [3] and HL7 Clinical Document Architecture [11]	Standards developed by ISO and CEN (Committee for Standardization) helps in achieving semantic interoper-	The need to represent the context in which clinical information needs to be shared is essential in healthcare	smartData Offshore Health Care application Development using PHP, Joomla, Drupal, Java

Table 1. (*Continued*)

Architecture	Features	Limitations	Models designed for Healthcare
(Generic reference models for representing clinical (EHR) data)	ability in the healthcare domain to fulfill the shared and secured healthcare scenario	domain and still remains a challenge in existing models.	

4   Standardization of Health Data

Vocabularies: Standards are obtained from a variety of efforts. Each department or facility of healthcare requires a standard vocabulary to be followed globally for successful exchange of heterogeneous health data with each other.

ISD: Vocabularies considered as standard for billing are the International classification of Disease (ISD) from World Health Organization (WHO) and the various country-specific versions.

NDC: The National Drug Code (NDC) is another standard for use within US pharmacy industry.

HDD: Healthcare Data Dictionary (HDD)[30] is designed to support the integration of coded data in the Clinical Data Repository (CDR). The content of HDD is cross-referenced to standard vocabularies, e.g. SNOMED CT, reference sources, e.g. UMLS, and classification schemes, e.g. the International Classification of Diseases, 9th Edition, Clinical Modification (ICD9CM).

CPT: Current Procedural Terminology (CPT) [34] is a comprehensive list of descriptive terms and codes published by the American Medical Association (AMA) and used for reporting diagnostic and therapeutic procedures and other medical services performed by physicians.

RxNorm: RxNorm[23] is a clinical drug nomenclature that provides standard names for clinical drugs (active ingredient, strength, and dose form) and for dose forms as administered.

Archetypes: Archetypes play a fundamental role for achieving interoperability in healthcare. Archetypes are chunks of declarative medical knowledge that are designed to capture maximally expressive and internationally reusable clinical information units. An archetype definition basically consists of three parts: descriptive data, constraint rules, and ontological definitions. The ISO EN 13606 and openEHR communities specify them using the Archetype Definition Language (ADL). Archetypes are based on conceptual structures of medical knowledge and provide standardized clinical contents. Archetypes are not linked a priority to any medical terminology but they can refer to multiple external medical classifications (e.g. SNOMED) from where controlled vocabularies are incorporated as labels of archetype elements.[22]

Message Exchange Standards

HL7: HL7 is a Standards Developing Organization accredited by the American National Standards Institute (ANSI) to author consensus-based standards representing a board view from healthcare system stakeholders. HL7 has compiled a collection of message formats and related clinical standards that define an ideal presentation of clinical information, and together the standards provide a framework in which data may be exchanged. The standard is based on the concept of application-to-application message exchange.

Digital Imaging and Communications in Medicine (DICOM): Messaging standard for digital images. A DICOM image consists of attributes which contains a multitude of image related information. It is based on client-server concept. DICOM is produced and managed by the DICOM standards committee, which consists of vendors, user organizations, government agencies, and trade associations.

5   Data Exchange Mechanisms

The content of the information exchange requests are unambiguously defined-: what is sent is the same as what is understood. A survey conducted by [8] gives an insight to various realistic scenarios prevalent in healthcare industry forfeiting availability of sophisticated and robust techniques of designing fine-tuned HIS. Securing data exchange between two systems is a very difficult task, considering a possible intrusion of an attacker on the flow of data. Enormous mechanisms exist catering to the requirements of sharing of data in between different systems.

Previously data could be stored in fixed format text files, or as bits of information with standard delimiting characters, commonly called CSV for "Comma Separated Values". Today, there is more dynamic format called XML (eXtensible Markup Language). Newer standards, like XML, are web-based and work in browsers, allowing for a more dynamic relationship with the data sets and less external programming. Number of XML-based metadata standards, including Encoded Archival Description (EAD), Metadata Object Description Schema (MODS), Metadata Authority Description Schema (MADS), Metadata Encoding and Transmission Standard (METS), Metadata for Images in XML (MIX), MPEG-21 Digital Item Declaration Language (DIDL), Open Archives Initiative Object Reuse and Exchange (OAI-ORE), Preservation Metadata Implementation Strategies (PREMIS) are developed for exchange of information between disparate systems.

But there are certain limitations to these standards. Web Services Description Language (WSDL) and XML Schema standards do not define how to move the documents between services, how to track the documents, or even how to interpret the documents. Efforts to exchange information employing XML incarnations of descriptive metadata standards such as Dublin Core [9] have fallen prey to a number of encoding and semantic inconsistencies.

6   Technical Interoperability Standards for EHR

Data standardization [17] refers to the use of the same set of codes to encode data throughout the system. Organizations face the challenge of exchanging, comparing, aggregating or integrating data among its multiple systems or facilities and also with external organizations.

HIPAA ASC X12 and National Council for Prescription Drug Programs (NCPDP) Batch Transaction Standard: HIPAA ASC X12 and NCPDP Batch Transaction Format provides practical guidelines and ensures consistent implementation throughout the industry of a file submission standard to be used between pharmacies and processors, or pharmacies, switches, and processors. (www.ncpdp.org)
Logical Observation Identifiers Names and Codes (LOINC): These identify test results or clinical observations uniquely. The observations consist of laboratories, clinical and administrative facilities. These codes are compatible with HL7 and SNOMED. (www.loinc.org)
Continuity of Care Document (CCD): In June 2005, the American Society for Testing and Materials (ASTM) unveiled the CCR (Continuity of Care) [33], data content and document standard for relaying a patient's core data set upon transfer. Health Level 7 (HL7), worked with the ASTM to harmonize the CCR with the CDA (Clinical Document Architecture), in 2000. The CDA enables the electronic transfer of multiple types of medical data from one healthcare institution to another. The CCD (Continuity of Care Document) is part of the Integrating the Healthcare Enterprise (IHE) IT Infrastructure Cross Enterprise Document Sharing (XDS) profiles for 2006 and 2007.

7   Conclusion

Enormous techniques and approaches lead to interoperability. This should ensure seamless sharing of data between organizations without any constraints or deficiencies. But, the reality is different. Availability of intelligent models supported by state-of-the-art mechanisms need to address various reality checks in healthcare domain that act as outliers while analyzing the suitability of these approaches for building a completely viable interoperable healthcare environment.

The study reveals that message passing standards does not cover all the real world aspects of communication. The messages are less understandable and contain more of Meta information than actual information. Talking with Indian perspective, there are very few hospitals that have Hospital Information Systems (HIS). Those who deal with EHRs talk in their own native format and have paid negligible attention towards standardization in terms of vocabularies, codes and data exchange with each other. Another major challenge is ensuring confidentiality, availability and integrity of records while creating multiple instances of the data across disparate organizations.

With all the standards and approaches at hand enabling EHR interoperability, there is still a need of customization and user-specific modeling to be designed according to the suitability of environment and its users, and at the same time, ensure standardization of interface and formats for facilitating data exchange between disparate systems. The benefits from exchanging consistent patient information must become more transparent, confidence must be nurtured that the data will be secure and confidential, organizations must trust those with whom they share information, and the sharing of information cannot be seen as in conflict with business or legal interests of the participants.

References

1. Levels of Information Systems Interoperability (LISI). C4ISR Architecture Working Group (1998)
2. Young, P., Chaki, N., Berzins, V., Luqi: Evaluation of middleware architectures in achieving system interoperability. In: 2003 Proceedings of the 14th IEEE International Workshop on Rapid Systems Prototyping, pp. 108–116 (2003)
3. George, Aphrodite, T., Michael, P.: Interoperability among Heterogeneous Services. In: IEEE International Conference in Services Computing, pp. 174–181 (2006)
4. GridWise™ Architecture Council. Interoperability Context-Setting Framework (March 2008)
5. OSGi Alliance, http://www.osgi.org
6. Open Systems: Designing and Developing Our Operational Interoperability, A Publication of the Defense Acquisition University (2010)
7. Heckmann, D., Schwarzkopf, E., Mori, J., Dengler, D., Kröner, A.: The User Model and Context Ontology GUMO revisited for future Web 2.0 Extensions (2007)
8. Bhartiya, S., Mehrotra, D.: Threats and Challenges to Security of Electronic Health Records. In: Singh, K., Awasthi, A.K., Mishra, R. (eds.) QSHINE 2013. LNICST, vol. 115, pp. 543–559. Springer, Heidelberg (2013)
9. Understanding Metadata, Copyright, National Information Standards Organization (2004), http://www.niso.org/publications/press/UnderstandingMetadata.pdf
10. Crista, O.: Techniques for Securing Data Exchange between a Database Server and a Client Program. In: 7th Tome 1st Fasc. Annals. Computer Science Series (2009)
11. Eve, R.: Enterprise Data Sharing: The New Data Virtualization Driver. Information Management (September 17, 2009), http://www.informationmanagement.com/infodirect/2009_139/enterprise_data_sharing_virtualization-10016067-1.html
12. Interoperability Guidelines, Oracle® Fusion Middleware, Concepts Guide for Oracle Infrastructure Web Services (January 2011), http://docs.oracle.com/cd/E17904_01/web.1111/e15184.pdf
13. Zaleski, J.: Integrating Device Data into the Electronic Medical Record. Wiley Publications
14. Harmon, B.: Healthcare Solutions, http://www.connectopensource.org/
15. Jin, L., Li, C., Mehrotra, S.: Efficient Record Linkage in Large Data Sets. In: SIGMOD 2007, Beijing, China, June 11-14, pp. 978–971 (2007); Copyright 2007 ACM 978-1-59593-686-8/07/0006

16. Stewart, B.A., Femandes, S., Rodriguez-Huertas, E., Landzberg, M.: A Preliminary look at duplicate testing associated with lack of electronic health record interoperability for transferred patients. Journal of the American Medical Informatics Associations 17(3), 341–344 (2010)

17. Grimson, J., Grimson, W., Berry, D., Stephens, G., Felton, E., Kalra, D., Toussaint, P., Weier, O.W.: A CORBA-Based Integration of Distributed Electronic Healthcare Records Using the Synapses Approach. IEEE Transactions on Information Technology in Biomedicine 2(3) (September 1998)

18. Ohe, K.: A hospital information system based on Common Object Request Broker Architecture (CORBA) for exchanging distributed medical objects–an approach to future environment of sharing healthcare information. Stud. Health Technol. Infor. 52(pt. 2), 962–964 (1998)

19. Rishel, W.: HL7 with CORBA and OLE: software components for healthcare. In: Proc. AMIA Annu. Fall Symp., pp. 95–99 (1996)

20. Henning, M.: The Rise and Fall of CORBA, June 1. ACMQueue (2006)

21. Menárguez-Tortosa, M., Fernández-Breis, J.T.: OWL-based Reasoning Methods for Validating Archetyped Clinical Knowledge. J. Biomed. Inform. (2013)

22. Nikolova, I., Angelova, G., Tcharaktchiev, D., Boytcheva, S.: Medical archetypes and information extraction templates in Automatic Processing of Clinical Narratives. In: Pfeiffer, H.D., Ignatov, D.I., Poelmans, J., Gadiraju, N. (eds.) ICCS 2013. LNCS, vol. 7735, pp. 106–120. Springer, Heidelberg (2013)

23. http://www.nlm.nih.gov/research/umls/rxnorm/index.html

24. Gelish, A.: Pacific Medical Network Project-pushing the edge of the envelope in information interoperability, pp. 37–42 (1998)

25. http://en.Wikipedia.org/wiki/HOSxP

26. Deftereos, S., Lambrinoudakis, C., Andriopoulos, P., Farmakis, D., Aessopos, A.: A Java-based Electronic Healthcare Record Software for Beta-thalassaemia. J. Med. Internet Res. 3(4), e33 (2001)

27. Puleston, C., Parsia, B., Cunningham, J., Rector, A.L.: Integrating Object-Oriented and Ontological Representations: A Case Study in Java and OWL. In: Sheth, A.P., Staab, S., Dean, M., Paolucci, M., Maynard, D., Finin, T., Thirunarayan, K. (eds.) ISWC 2008. LNCS, vol. 5318, pp. 130–145. Springer, Heidelberg (2008)

28. Zhang, J.K., Xu, W., Ewins, D.: System Interoperability Study for Healthcare Information System with Web Services. Journal of Computer Science 3(7), 1549–3636 (2007) ISSN 1549-3636 © 2007 Science Publications

29. A New Approach Expanding SOA in Healthcare Eric Leader, VP Technology Architecture and Product Management, Carefx (July 2010)

30. Lau, L.M.: Towards Data Interoperability: Practical Issues in Terminology Implementation and Mapping. In: Clinical Vocabulary Mapping Method Institute, 77th AHIMA Convention and Exhibit (October 2005)

31. Spackman, K.: An examination of OWL and the requirements of a large health care terminology (2006)

32. Perumal, T., Ramli, A.R., Leong, C.Y., Mansor, S., Samsudin, K.: Interoperability for Smart Home Environment Using Web Services. International Journal of Smart Home 2(4) (October 2008)

33. Data Standards, Data Quality, and Interoperability. Appendix A: Data Standards Resource. Journal of AHIMA 78(2) (February 2007)

34. Current Procedural Terminology, Excerpt from Current Procedural Terminology, published by the American Medical Association (2013)

Visual Data Discovery to Support Patient Care

Jihong Zeng[1] and John Zhang[2]

[1] School of Management, New York Institute of Technology,
Old Westbury, New York, USA
jzeng@nyit.edu
[2] New York City Health & Hospitals Corporation, New York, USA
john.zhang@nychhc.org

Abstract. Adopting electronic health records fuel exponential data growth. However, more data doesn't necessarily lead to more information unless you have an efficient tool to translate massive data into actionable insights in real time and in a cost-effective manner. This paper is a preliminary study which introduces a new breed of data discovery technology and its value as emerging differentiator from traditional business intelligence, especially in the usability perspective. We present an exemplary case of using QlikView for clinical report dashboard. Physicians and care providers explore patient populations, data patterns, answer questions spontaneously, and forge new drill paths through data volume of millions of rows. Initial evaluation result is promising and indicates visual data discovery tool empowers end users with intuitive and interactive experience, rapid deployment, customizable ad-hoc questions and answers. The next step will be integration with data governance, advanced statistics, predictive modeling and thorough user evaluation with subject matter experts including clinical and IT staff.

Keywords: visual data discovery, business intelligence, interactive visualization, clinical dashboard.

1   Introduction

Healthcare industry is in transformation in order to provide patients with world class quality of care at low cost. Healthcare provider reimbursements will increasingly be tied to quality metrics and patient outcomes under healthcare reform. The Health Information Technology for Economic and Clinical Health Act (HITECH 2009) allocated billions of dollars to incentivize doctors and hospitals to adopt electronic health records (EHRs) [1]. Digital health files fuel exponential data growth. However, more data doesn't necessarily lead to more insight. Back in 2006, Palmer used an analogy between data and oil in his blogs. He stated that "Data is just like crude. It's valuable, but if unrefined it cannot really be used. It has to be changed into gas, plastic, chemicals, etc to create a valuable entity that drives profitable activity; so must data be broken down, analyzed for it to have value" [2]. Therefore, healthcare providers need efficient tools to translate massive data into meaningful, actionable insight for the

D. Zeng et al. (Eds.): ICSH 2013, LNCS 8040, pp. 66–70, 2013.

front-line clinicians in real time and in a cost-effective manner in support of better patient care outcomes and quality improvement.

In this paper, we describe the challenge and need for an efficient data discovery tool in a large healthcare provider organization in Section 2. Then we introduce a new breed of visual data discovery technology and high level application architecture in Section 3. We then discuss a use case on clinical data discovery and analytics proto-type dashboard with QlikView in Section 4. The paper concludes in Section 5 with a discussion of the next step for further thorough user evaluation.

2   Challenge and Motivation

Previous studies confirm the positive impact of health information technology components on patient care outcomes. However, its usability is of vital importance for system adoption and sustained use. As summarized by Dorr et al after review over a hundred articles and systems on patient care, ease of use and respect for care providers' time constraints are important usability considerations [3].

Here is the real world challenge at one of the largest healthcare providers in the US. During the past decades, this healthcare provider has been an industry leader in the usage of electronic medical record (EMR) systems and was one of the first providers in the country to implement an EMR. Patient data from operational database are ported to Oracle data warehouse through nightly batch processing in the back-end. Oracle Discoverer is the front-end tool for queries and reports. However, majority of the traditional business intelligence (BI) reports rely on tabular data displays, which don't easily reveal patterns or trends, nor effectively provide one holistic view of patient information throughout the care episode. Queries and reports are pre-determined to specific requests. In addition, lengthy development cycle for new report cannot meet the business need. During month end report generating period, users could experience long waiting time for the database query due to degraded performance of the data warehouse. The front-line clinicians need to focus on patient rather than data. With shift to pay-for-performance and increasing regulatory compliance requirements, the provider organization is in serious demand for a more efficient and effective tool to help transform terabytes of collected data into actionable insight.

3   Visual Data Discovery Application Architecture

Traditional BI data presentation methods require conscious thinking. However, cognitive function of human brain is slower and less efficient. As pointed out by data visualization expert Stephen Few that "approximately 70% of the body's sense receptors reside in our eyes" [4]. For the human brain, visual perception is fast and efficient. Data visualization takes advantage of our most powerful sense, helps us think and communicate. A picture is worth a thousand words. Picture of data can help make the invisible visible. Rind et al provided a comprehensive survey on the state-of-art of information visualization systems for EHRs and suggested that EHR vendors have great potential to apply innovative visual methods to support clinical decision-making and research [5].

Filling the void by traditional BI products and becoming mainstream, visual data discovery tools provide highly interactive graphic user interface, enable users to develop and refine views and analyses of data on the fly using search terms. According to Sommer et al [6], they have the following key characteristics:

- **Agile**: proprietary data structure that minimizes reliance on predefined business intelligence metadata. Rapid application development and deployment to meet business need
- **Performance**: in-memory database and analytics engine that boosts query performance. Enable users interact with data on the fly
- **Ease of Use**: intuitive interface that enables users to explore data without much training. Target business users as a self-service BI rather than IT professionals

QlikView is the leading visual data discovery software by QlikTech [6]. Based on its in-memory data associative architecture, QlikView enables users gain unexpected insights by understanding how data is associated. For example, when user selects a data point in a field, no queries are initiated. Instead, all other fields associated instantaneously filter themselves based on the user selection. It enables users to answer questions like: What has happened? Why did it happen? What will happen next? What's the next best action?

In response to the business challenge, the large healthcare provider organization developed new clinical reporting dashboards using QlikView after proof-of-concept evaluation. Data from various sources are extracted in QlikView Data (QVD) file format by QlikView ETL application. The front-end QlikView dashboard application aggregates data from multiple intermediate QVD files. With the associative data architecture, QlikView is able to achieve data compression ratio 100:1 for the dataset used in this study, making high performance interactive, visual data discovery on the dataset of 59 million rows, 1.4 billion records. Access to QlikView dashboard is controlled and managed by IT security management. User authentication and authorization are integrated with Windows active directory service architecture. Users access the QlikView dashboard applications through standard web browser. Only developers use QlikView Desktop Edition for application development and enhancement.

4   Results and Discussion

With its highly interactive, ease-of-use graphical interface, QlikView helps create a patient centered view by integrating information from multiple data sources including EMR data warehouse, chronic disease registry and provider panel management system. Figure 1 illustrates some sample screen captures of the QlikView dashboard for integrated patient panel management system. The dashboard includes key performance indicators such as percentage of patients visiting their assigned primary care providers or alternative providers, top 10 providers for continuity of care, etc.

The continuity of primary care is important for reducing hospital readmissions, especially for patients with chronic diseases. The dashboard content and display update dynamically based on user selections by clicking filters such as facility, age group, year, month. The dashboard also provides advanced visualization such as trellis charts and animated bubble charts time series to help compare performance across multiple care facilities and illustrate performance improvement over time. The dashboard also enables users to drill down to granular level detail data by clicking on individual item on a summary report.

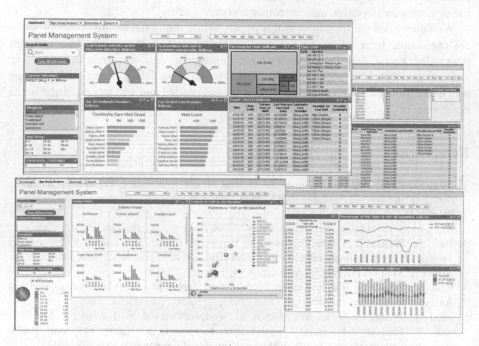

Fig. 1. QlikView Dashboard for Integrated Patient Panel Management System

Initial evaluation result indicates visual data discovery empowers end users with visual, intuitive and interactive end user experience, rapid deployment, customizable ad-hoc questions and answers. Clinicians and care providers explore patient populations, data patterns, answer questions spontaneously, and forge new drill paths through data volume of millions of rows in search for insight. The new solution platform also provides a single consolidated view of performance across the organization. This enables hospital administrators to monitor performance at all its care facilities, identify problems through trend and pattern, and find root-causes through drill down into granular level data, such as drill-down to facility level and individual provider or patient level, for process improvement strategy and policy.

5   Conclusion

This paper introduces the emerging visual data discovery tool and presents its value for healthcare providers in transforming massive data into valuable information and insight. Positive feedback is received from clinicians and care administrators for pilot use cases at a large healthcare provider organization. Visual data discovery enables end users to navigate and interact without limit of predefined data drill paths or using preconfigured reports. It helps make the invisible visible and helps clinicians focus on patients rather than data. It could also be a revenue enhancing tool through better imbursement by improved care outcomes and care quality.

We understand the limitation of this paper. While the initial results from our study are promising, there are many potential enhancements in the future. This includes integrating visual data discovery tool with enterprise data governance, interfacing with advanced statistic package, and adding predictive modeling. Additional thorough user evaluation with subject matter experts is also needed and will be conducted in the next step.

References

1. Blumenthal, D.: Implementation of the Federal Health Information Technology Initiative. New England Journal of Medicine 365, 2426–2431 (2011)
2. Palmer, M.:
   http://ana.blogs.com/maestros/2006/11/data_is_the_new.html
3. Dorr, D., Bonner, L., Cohen, A., Shoai, R., Perrin, R., Chaney, E., Young, A.: Informatics Systems to Promote Improved Care for Chronic Illness: A Literature Review. Journal of the American Medical Informatics Association 14, 156–163 (2007)
4. Few, S.: Now You See It: Simple Visualization Techniques for Quantitative Analysis. Analytics Press, Oakland (2009)
5. Rind, A., Wang, T., Aigner, W., Miksch, S., Wongsuphasawat, K., Plaisant, C., Shneiderman, B.: Interactive Information Visualization to Explore and Query Electronic Health Records. Foundations and Trends in Human-Computer Interaction 5, 207–298 (2013)
6. Sommer, D., Sallam, R., Richardson, J.: Emerging Technology Analysis: Visualization-Based Data Discovery Tools. Gartner Publication ID Number G00213778 (2011)
7. QlikTech, http://www.qlikview.com

DiabeticLink: A Health Big Data System
for Patient Empowerment and Personalized Healthcare

Hsinchun Chen[1], Sherri Compton[1], and Owen Hsiao[2]

[1] University of Arizona, Artificial Intelligence Lab, Tucson, Arizona
hchen@eller.arizona.edu, scompton@email.arizona.edu
[2] National Taiwan University, Health Information Research, Taipei, Taiwan
owen.w.hsiao@gmail.com

Abstract. Ever increasing rates of diabetes and healthcare costs have focused our attention on this chronic disease to provide a health social media system to serve multi-national markets. Our *DiabeticLink* system has been developed in both the US and Taiwan markets, addressing the needs of patients, caretakers, nurse educators, physicians, pharmaceutical company and researchers alike to provide features that encourage social connection, data sharing and assimilation and educational opportunities. Some important features *DiabeticLink* offers include diabetic health indicator tracking, electronic health record (EHR) search, social discussion and Q&A forums, health information resources, diabetic medication side effect reporting, healthy eating recipes and restaurant recommendations. We utilize advanced data, text and web mining algorithms and other computational techniques that are relevant to healthcare decision support and cyber-enabled patient empowerment.

Keywords: Health Big Data, Diabetes, health social media, data mining.

1 Introduction

The World Health Organization (WHO) estimates that 346 million people worldwide have diabetes and that this number will double by 2030. In the US, 18.8 million people have been diagnosed with diabetes and nearly 7 million people remain undiagnosed [1]. The cost of diabetes in the US is expected to be near $245 billion for diagnosed cases in 2012; medical expenditures of Diabetics' tend to be 2.3 times higher than for non-diabetics [2]. As discouraging as these numbers are, Diabetes is very much a disease that can be prevented or delayed with improved lifestyle and diet choices. However, the US healthcare tradition does not include a strong history of prioritizing proactive prevention, management and patient empowerment programs to stem a significant failure to motivate people to take charge of their lifestyle and health decisions. Limitations in healthcare access, delivery and education solutions leave many patients wanting for direction relating to proper disease self-management strategies.

We believe these factors will force many patients to seek a more personalized, proactive and adaptive healthcare delivery system to better manage and control their

D. Zeng et al. (Eds.): ICSH 2013, LNCS 8040, pp. 71–83, 2013.

disease outcomes. We also see a space in the healthcare delivery market for newer tools for patients and informatics and clinical researchers and educators such as those being developed by our project, the patient portal *DiabeticLink,* currently being developed in parallel by US and Taiwanese teams for release in each region.

2   Health Big Data and Patient Support Review

Today's healthcare has become cost-prohibitive for many and suffers substantially from medical errors and waste [3]. An often-cited reference is the 1998 Institute of Medicine report, which estimated that preventable medical errors lead to as many as 98,000 deaths per year in the United States [4]. In Anderson & Markovich [5], it was reported that the U.S. spends $1.7 trillion annually (16% of GDP) on healthcare, yet produces significantly lower health outcomes than many other developed countries. Many new government initiatives have been started recently to address this continuing problem and improve healthcare-related outcomes. For example, President Obama's $787 billion federal stimulus package was announced in 2009. The HITECH Act for healthcare information technology (IT) stipulates that healthcare entities in the U.S. need to use IT to fix ingrained problems, with $19 billion in 2011 and a total of $50 billion allocated to this effort over the next 5 years. In January 2009, China's government announced a plan to spend more than $120 billion on the first phase of a 10-year overhaul of the healthcare system [6]. In academia there has also been significant recent interest in adopting and advancing IT for effective healthcare. The 2009 National Research Council report on "Computational Technology for Effective Health Care" suggests an overarching research grand challenge of developing "patient-centered cognitive support." It also points out several representative research challenges for the IT community, including: virtual patient modeling, healthcare automation, healthcare data sharing and collaboration, and healthcare data management at scale. A major research goal of these programs is to develop trusted healthcare systems that offer relevant decision support to clinicians and patients and offer "just in time, just for me" advice at the point of care.

In a recent research commentary article by Wactlar, Pavel and Barkis entitled "Can Computer Science Save Healthcare?" [7], the authors discuss ways that computer science (or more generally IT) research could help to resolve some of the healthcare crises in America. They propose a program of research and development along four technology thrusts to enable this vision: (1) creating an interoperable, digital infrastructure of universal health data and knowledge, (2) utilizing diverse data to provide automated and augmented insight, discovery, and evidence-based health and wellness decision support, (3) a cyber-based empowering of patients and healthy individuals to play a substantial role in their own health and treatment, and (4) monitoring and assisting individuals with intelligent systems: sensors, devices and robotics, to maintain function and independence.

Thrust areas 2 and 3, *healthcare decision support* and *cyber-enabled patient empowerment*, are of particular relevance to our proposed project. Given the growing numbers of electronic health records (EHR), results of clinical trials, high-throughput genomic research findings, the biomedical research literature, and even health-related social data, healthcare is entering the realm of "Health Big Data." Advanced data mining, machine learning, natural language processing, and data visualization research, carefully developed with clinical consideration in the diagnosis, treatment, and patient care cycle, are critically needed. Moreover, patients and their families are and should be full healthcare decision partners. Patients who actively participate in their healthcare have better outcomes and a perceived quality of life that is better than those who do not [8]. Patient empowerment can be supported by new communication and sensor technologies, decision support systems, and health social media tools.

Likewise the Taiwanese government is promoting the development a cloud platform to meet the following requirements to support its healthcare industry: (1) construction of shared platforms for Big Data, (2) development of massively distributed processing technology, and (3) development of tools or platforms that can produce value-added health informatics applications. Along with large multinationals such as IBM and Microsoft, local companies Wistron and Datacom Technology Corporation continue to increase investment in big data analytics solutions to improve healthcare service delivery and preventive consumer healthcare.

In both regions, diabetic-centric resources for disease management and education are either lacking or limited and leave many patients wanting for direction relating to proper disease self-monitoring strategies. Traditional healthcare solutions do not tend to include strong proactive preventive initiatives or disease management and patient empowerment programs to stem a significant failure to motivate people to take charge of their lifestyle and health decisions. In the US, soaring costs, tightening budgets and 50 million uninsured Americans help fuel the demand for inexpensive, on-demand resources such as patient portals like *DiabeticLink* can deliver.

3   Diabetes Market Review

3.1   Diabetes Patients as Users

With diabetes affecting approximately 8% of the population of the United States and Taiwan (25.8 million and 2 million people respectively) the development of patient-oriented social networks supported via health social media and mobile technologies (e.g., web forums, mobile devices, micro-blogging) for different patient communities can potentially help with more proactive and timely patient care and produce better long-term health outcomes. Health social media sites such as DailyStrength and PatientsLikeMe provide unique research opportunities in healthcare decision support and patient empowerment, especially for chronic diseases such as Diabetes, Parkinson's disease, Alzheimer's disease, and cancer. Internet usage is high in both countries, estimated at 80% and 72% for the US and Taiwan respectively, contributing to the high volume of traffic on health social medial sites. Initial estimates put the expected number of patient users in Taiwan at over 1 million per month.

Established diabetes social media sites with community forums and other social features to connect patients and encourage the sharing of information exist in both English and Chinese. Tables 1 and 2 outline the sites available in both languages. These sites provide content-rich patient postings and profiles, valuable for extracting symptom, disease and treatment (SDT) and patient sentiment information. Based on our deep web spidering research and systems experience [9] we have collected over 3.3 million postings in English and over 2 million postings in Chinese. Whereas all of the English sites allow for two-way communication between site members on discussion forum boards, *DiabeticLink* is the first patient portal to provide such an interactive platform to exchange disease information and experience. Similar to other diabetes social media sites, there are three main types of diabetic patients who would use our site: Type 1, Type 2 and Gestational. "Pre-Diabetics" – those who show likelihood to develop Type 2, or "Adult Onset" diabetes – would also benefit from using our product. Although each group may have slightly different goals in managing their condition, *DiabeticLink* is relevant to the entire population of diabetics and pre-diabetic patients.

Table 1. Comparison of system features for diabetes social media sites in English. The main competitors to *DiabeticLink* in the US are dLife.com, the American Diabetes Association (diabetes.org) and Diabetes.co.uk. Our innovative Aggregated Forums, Drug Side Effect reporting, EHR Search and mobile-to-web integrated diabetes tracking modules make *DiabeticLink* truly competitive in the healthcare social media space.

	DiabeticLink	dLife IT'S YOUR DIABETES LIFE!	American Diabetes Association.	Diabetes.co.uk the global diabetes community
Aggregated Forums	✓	No	No	No
Adverse Drug Reactions	✓	No	No	No
EHR Search tool	✓	No	No	No
Portal Tracking app integrated with Mobile	✓	No	No	(Portal tracking, but no integration)
Mobile Tracking app (Glucose, weight, A1c, medications, food/activity log, etc)	✓	(Glucose only; search recipes; Q&A)	(ADA journals only)	No
Community Forums; Social Connectivity; Meal Plans; Food & Fitness Guides; Diabetes Guides and Health Information	✓	✓	✓	✓

Table 2. Comparison of system features for diabetes sites in Taiwan. The main competitors in Chinese are Formosa Diabetes Care Foundation (dmcare.org.tw), bs.tnbz.com, and the Diabetes Association of the Republic of China (diabetes.org.tw). The Chinese language market is much less developed; therefore, our social connectivity features, integrated diabetes tracking, National Health Insurance Data query capabilities and healthy recipe and restaurant search will put us at the forefront of a complete and innovative online social health system.

	DiabeticLink		甜蜜家园 bbs.tnbz.com	
Community Forums; Social Connectivity & Personal Blogs	✓	No	(Online forum only)	No
FDA ADE & Drug Search	✓	No	No	No
National Health Insurance Data (NHI) Query	✓	No	No	No
Healthy Recipes & Healthy Restaurant Search	✓	(General dining guides only)	(Individual users' posts in forum discussions only)	No
Portal Tracking App Integrated with Mobile	✓	No	No	No
Diabetes Guides & Health Information	✓	✓	✓	✓

3.2 Other Users

Caretakers. These users may be family members or friends who wish to learn more about the disease and its complications in order to better support their loved one. Caretakers can benefit from seeking support on discussion forums, reading educational materials or using interactive tools to supplement the fundamentals of their understanding of this complex disease.

Nurse Educators. Often providing the patient's first introduction to their new condition, Nurse Educators benefit greatly from an accessible resource at their fingertips. Initial Nurse feedback indicated that they have only one hour to run through the gamut of information a diabetic needs to make life-changing decisions for keeping the disease under control. This group of consumers benefit from being able to sit with a new diabetic in the clinic and go through a website such as *DiabeticLink* in order to give order to the myriad of choices each patient will face. The nurses are very enthusiastic about the value they see *DiabeticLink* brings to their patients.

Physicians. Much like Nurse Educators, physicians are short on time to get many new concepts through to a newly-diagnosed diabetic. This group also sees how the *DiabeticLink* tools and resources saves time and gives meaning to the vast knowledge base that make up the proactive diabetic's undertaking.

Researchers. The potential for researchers to gain knowledge through data-mined electronic health records (EHR) is much anticipated. EHR can capture potentially more complete details of a patient's symptoms, treatments and outcomes than other self-reporting methods (which are available on other sites like PatientsLikeMe.com). Trends can be captured on an anonymous and large-scale manner, benefitting diabetics and researchers alike.

Pharmacists. *DiabeticLink's* aggregation of the FDA's Adverse Drug Effects data and patient discussion forum comments on drugs aids pharmacists in the field in gaining real-time patient reactions to drugs and their interactions.

4   System Functionalities

The current project involves building a diabetes patient portal called *DiabetickLink*. This portal implements the advanced algorithms and techniques developed in the AI Lab and offers a robust, easy-to-use system that collects patient data and experiences while he/she interacts and engages with *DiabetickLink* and its community. This collection of interactions, data and relationships build by the site's users is then available to researchers to learn more about patients' disease management efforts. There are four main types of features being developed.

Unique Patient Intelligence Tools. For manipulating patient information to reveal relationships between lifestyle, treatment and outcome factors in an easy-to-understand online format. Data mining large EHR datasets and social media content presents users with new methods and services for preventive interventions. Healthcare providers also see the value of being able to show patient trends in successful disease management. For example, by viewing other patients' improvements after going on insulin, the user may be more inclined to make a life-enhancing decision to go on insulin as well.

Disease Management Tools. Tracking of critical diabetes disease parameters (e.g. Blood Glucose, Blood Pressure, HbA1c, etc.), food/nutrition, physical activity levels, medication and insulin dosage is imperative to enabling patients to monitor their health and disease progression. Diabetics often complain about the time-consuming process of tracking important health and lifestyle indicators. Our solution saves time and improves compliance by providing a simple, easy-to-use platform with convenient web portal and mobile integration and report-generating capabilities. We also clearly track carbohydrates to insulin needs for which no active application is currently available.

Social Connection. Social forums for patient discussions and member profiles provide a safe and anonymous platform to share treatment management questions, experiences, successes and challenges. Users can benefit from readily-available and critical online social support throughout their journey. Our product is innovative in that it allows users to search for similar patients across multiple discussion forums, not just one at a time. Patient data protection of user data is of highest priority.

Education. Up-to-date health information, videos and news articles are sourced from credible diabetes sites (American Diabetes Association, NIH, etc.). All users benefit from being able to remain on our site to meet all of their disease management needs, including the features mentioned above.

4.1   US Version Features

Social Media Platform: Discussion Forums, Member Profiles, Activity, Friending, Following. The goal of this module is to allow patient to connect to others and share their experience and/or offer support to others. Visitors are encouraged to register, create an online profile (which can be anonymous), update his/her status, add photos, write a blog, invite and add friends, find others with similar interests, post questions or provide support to others in the discussion forums. Such features are a mainstay on the health social media sites we have highlighted previously.

Tracking Diabetes and Lifestyle Risk Factors (Blood Glucose, HbA1c, Blood Pressure, Food, Activity, etc.). Patients will find an easy-to-use interface that helps the user manage his/her diabetes by tracking important measures of health and there-by creating a digital representation of the disease. Entries can be added easily and summaries and dashboards display clear graphical results to be viewed or printed out for healthcare provider or patient use. One particularly innovative feature is the display of multiple measurements side-by-side to better illustrate trends and areas to improve or better manage. Data can be entered via a mobile device which is synched with the web application to increase monitoring compliance and convenience.

FDA ADE & Drug Search. The Federal Drug Administration (FDA) Adverse Event Reporting System (FAERS) database is analyzed and visualized to simplify the patient's search for post-marketing reports of side effects and other safety concerns. This database contains information on adverse event and medication error reports submitted voluntarily to the FDA by mostly physicians and consumers. Patients can search by a particular drug name, by a safety concern (or side effect), related conditions that co-exist with diabetes (e.g. hypertension) or by comparing two drugs. Results of top safety concerns by drug and the timeline showing the frequency of submitted adverse event reports are displayed. Searches can be performed on the raw FAERS data files as well. Phase two development of this module includes patient comments data mined from social media content, showing sentiment for each drug (opinions and experiences) and any safety concerns experienced.

EHR Search. We have procured an EHR dataset from MS (anonymized) General Hospital in Taiwan which contains nearly 2.5 million records for nearly 893,000 patients. Our plan is to identify critical symptom-disease-treatment associations based on patient demographics and disease stage information. Such a "scenario-based" data mining approach allows us to consider the rich healthcare context that is unique to each patient subgroup. Our first steps include analyzing and identifying health relevant data fields and representations in EHR for subsequent data and text analysis. Our tool clearly shows how better lifestyle choices lead to better disease outcomes, serving as a useful educational tool to patients, clinicians and researchers alike.

Multi-forum Search. This module allows patient to conduct a search across many forums at once, where currently no such search is available. So far we have only implemented selected benchmark algorithms for health social media analysis. We hope to continue our algorithm development with the proposed techniques in the next few years. We anticipate significant values from such analytical results for patient support and empowerment. We have collected more than 3 million individual posts, including 662,000 postings from diabetesforum.com, 600,000 postings from diabetesdaily.com, 280,000 from tudiabetes.org and 270,000 from diabetes.co.uk. The contents include health-relevant problems, treatment and outcome information and rich community interaction data. Our analysis and interpretation is based on sentiment analysis of healthcare contents expressed in health social media sites. Based on free-text forum discussions of many members in a health subgroup, we hope to represent the individual and aggregate attitude and response towards specific symptoms, diseases, and treatments (that are extracted from CRFs techniques mentioned previously) in the community. We also plan to utilize several temporal text mining approaches to take into account the dynamic nature of patient discussion forums.

4.2   Taiwan Version Features

Health Information Resources. In this module, DiabeticLink provides various diabetes related information to the users, including the basic diabetic related knowledge, latest diabetes related news and research reports. In our beta version, we provide a number of 341 quality traditional Chinese articles to our users. We collected our contents not only from prestigious Taiwanese health authorities and organizations such as Bureau of Health Promotion, Department of Health and Diabetes association of the Republic of China, but also from our alliances with other credible Taiwanese health media such as United Daily News and Healthnews.com.tw.

Healthy Recipes and Restaurant Search. In these two modules, we provide a total of 652 health-oriented recipes and restaurant to our users in our beta version. These recipes and restaurant information allow our users to have the knowledge of how to prepare healthy meals and where to dine out on healthy diets for diabetes patients. In the recipe module, we have not only provided the standard recipe information to our users, but also the nutrient charts (including glucose and calorie) so that our users could make quick calculation for their calorie and glucose intakes each meal. In our restaurant module, we have listed the suggest dishes from each restaurant so that our users know the most popular dishes for other health concern patrons. We have collected our content from numerous prestigious Taiwanese health authorities including Food and Drug Administration, Department of Health; Bureau of Health Promotion, Department of Health and Bureaus of Health of Taipei city.

National Health Insurance Data (NHI) Query. One of the special features that we have in *DiabeticLink*'s Taiwan site is the module called NHI Data Output. The goal of this module is to answer some of the most frequently asked questions which the diabetes patients and their caretakers may have with statistical reports extracted from the Taiwanese National Health Insurance database. We have sorted the questions into the following four categories: prevalence of Diabetes in Taiwan, Out-patient Related Questions, Inpatient Related Questions, and Medication Related Questions. Users are asked to choose the questions which they are interested in and to enter their personal information such as gender, and age. This data is used to query our database to request the corresponding statistics from the Taiwanese National Health Insurance database and show the results to our users.

In this module, we use the sampling data of two million people between 2000 and 2009 from Taiwan's National Health Insurance Database to form the statistical reports that we show to our users by utilizing SAS version 9.1. We have followed procedures as per Chang and his colleagues' work [10] in 2012 in order to produce our results. The NHI database contains the following information: ambulatory, and hospitalization care files, including dates of visits, medical care facilities; patients' sex, date of birth; the three to five diagnoses (ICD-9-CM); and the medical expenses for each visit from all medical care institutions under contract to the Bureau of National Health Insurance (BHNI) of Taiwan. Patients were classified as having diabetes and included in the analysis if they had at least one diabetes admission code or $>=3$ outpatient codes within 365 calendar days. To avoid accumulation of misdiagnosis, we used the selection method described for each year.

5   User Study and Feedback

We have interviewed several diabetes patients and physicians for user study purposes in both the US and Taiwan market. In these interviews we received positive feedback for providing diet advice and information regarding complications to the patients. Diabetes Nurse Educators in the US are very enthusiastic about having a resource which provides health information and educational tools to assist their education sessions with newly diagnosed diabetics who must learn about effective disease management. In our interviews with Taiwanese physicians, Dr. Lee Hong-Yuan, a physician from National Taiwan University Hospital (NTUH), pointed out that most of the patients wanted to understand how to manage their blood glucose from their diets during the outpatient appointments. We received similar feedback in our interview with Mr. Chang Quan-Lai, the president of the NTUT diabetes patient support group. In the interview, Mr. Chang expressed that most diabetes patients would like to know what they should eat and how for their diets. Also, Mr. Chang pointed out that he thinks it is also important for diabetes patients to pay attention to the information regarding complication since the complications are irreversible.

We have also received positive feedback from the patients regarding our online forum module. Patients in the US have responded favorably to our easy-to-use diabetes tracking module and its convenient mobile integration with the web application. In our interview with Mr. Chang, he pointed out that the online forum module provides patients a platform to exchange useful information and experiences in real time. We plan to conduct focus group studies with not only diabetes patients and their care takers but also the general public who wish to learn more about diabetes after we launch the beta version in order to get users' feedback regarding our UI design, and the usefulness of our contents to help us improve our websites.

As a capstone effort of our research program, we plan to conduct a multi-year, multi-stage field study to examine the usefulness and impact of our proposed techniques and health social media contents for patient support and empowerment. Our field study explores the usefulness and effectiveness of our *DiabeticLink* portal system and its cloud-based mobile delivery.

6   Sample System Screenshots

Development of *DiabeticLink* continues in both the US and Taiwan. This section presents sample screenshots of modules for each version for comparison. Where simultaneous development of a module occurs in the US and Taiwan, samples are taken from both and compared in one figure (Figures 1 and 2). Figures 3, 4, and 5 show two screenshots of the same module currently unique to the region. The Tracking and ADE modules will be adapted for the Taiwan market in the near future.

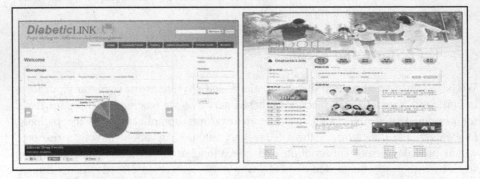

Fig. 1. *DiabeticLink* homepage of US version (left) and Taiwan version (right). The homepages offer an overview of each site's content and activity, and invites users to explore and become registered member. Registration unlocks social features such as discussion forum posting and member profile creation.

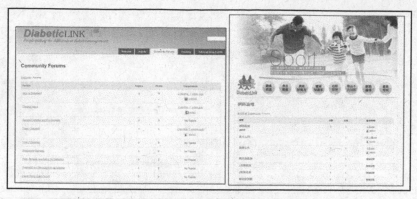

Fig. 2. *DiabeticLink* patient discussion forums screenshot of US version (top) and Taiwan version (bottom). The community forums encourage patient Q&A and social support activities. Pre-defined topics guide users to relevant subject matter, including Newly Diagnosed and Type 1 and 2; a summary of recent, popular and new topics enable the user to stay abreast of recent forum activity. New topics can be added as required.

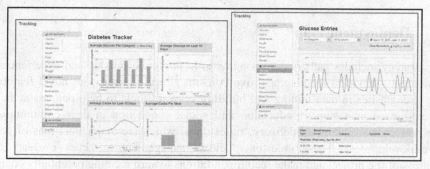

Fig. 3. Tracking module dashboard summary of patient data screenshot (left) and Blood Glucose summary display (right). Users can track, display, edit, print and view summaries of blood glucose, carbohydrates, medications, insulin, physical activity, blood pressure, body weight and Hemoglobin A1c levels. Varied time categories (e.g. before breakfast, after lunch) are provided to create more accurate summaries as well as international measurement units to simplify recording activities.

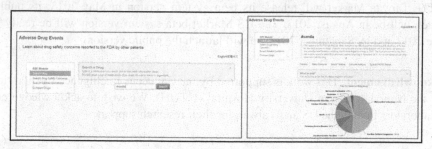

Fig. 4. Adverse Drug Event search (left) and results (right) for Avandia. We data mine the US FDA's Adverse Event Reporting System (FAERS) to search and compare diabetic medications for side effects and safety concerns related to diabetic conditions and display results in a simple interface.

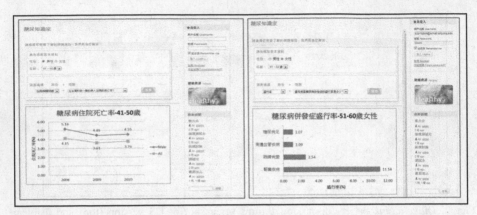

Fig. 5. NHI Data query output. Patients can search a NHI database to determine statistics for the rate of diabetes and answers to frequently asked inpatient/outpatient and medication questions. Search criteria utilize the patient's own demographic information, providing a more personalized and relevant results.

7   Deployment Plan

Our strategy includes gathering a strong team in proven leadership and experience to implement our vision for a competitive consumer health portal with novel features. Our strength lies in data mining and building relevant tools to help patients achieve better disease management, education and social connection in their communities. The project has established delivery 'milestones' which are major iterations of software development. These milestones allow management to better evaluate the progress of the project and make recommendations toward meeting potentially changing business needs. Project results will continue to be tracked and measured against these iterative milestone dates as the project progresses. An iteration presents an improvement in features and functionality which can be objectively tested and proved. Each release will involve extensive user studies and focus group studies to gain feedback on improving user interface and layout.

The Taiwan Market will release its beta system version in May 2013; its public launch will be in August 2013. The US Market beta system version will be ready in June 2013 and by September 2013 we will launch the public version.

Acknowledgement. This work is supported by the Caduceus Intelligence Corporation and the National Taiwan University Hospital (NTUH). We wish to acknowledge our collaborators in both the US and Taiwan for their research support.

References

1. Center for Disease Control and Prevention: National Diabetes Fact Sheet (2011), http://www.cdc.gov/diabetes/pubs/pdf/ndfs_2011.pdf
2. American Diabetes Association: Economic Costs of Diabetes in the United States in 2012. Diabetes Care 36, 1033–1046 (2013)
3. National Research Council, Computational Technology for Effective Health Care: Immediate Steps and Strategic Directions. The National Academies Press, Washington, DC (2009)
4. Institute of Medicine, To Err Is Human: Building a Safer Health System. National Academy Press, Washington, DC (2000)
5. Anderson, G., Markovich, P.: Multinational Comparisons of Health Systems Data. The Commonwealth Fund, New York (2009)
6. Fairclough, G.: In China, Rx for Ailing Health System. Wall Street Journal (October 15, 2009)
7. Wactlar, H., Pavel, M., Barkis, W.: Can Computer Science Save Healthcare? IEEE Intelligent Systems (September/October 2011)
8. Bandura, A.: Self-efficacy in health functioning. In: Ayers, S., et al. (eds.) Cambridge Handbook of Psychology, Health & Medicine, 2nd edn. Cambridge University Press, New York (2007)
9. Fu, T., Abbasi, A., Chen, H.: A Focused Crawler for Dark Web Forums. Journal of the American Society for Information Science and Technology 61(6) (2010)
10. Chang, T.J., Jiang, Y.D., Chang, C.H., Chung, C.H., Yu, N.C., Chuang, L.M.: Accountability, utilization and providers for diabetes management in Taiwan, 2000–2009: An analysis of the National Health Insurance database. Journal of the Formosan Medical Association (2012)

A Biofeedback System for Mobile Healthcare Based on Heart Rate Variability

Meijun Xiong, Rui He, Lianying Ji, and Jiankang Wu

Sensor Networks and Application Research Center (SNARC)
University of Chinese Academy Sciences
Beijing, China
{xmjdream,henryalps,jilianying,jiankangwu}@gmail.com

Abstract. Heart rate variability biofeedback provides a new technique for the evaluation of autonomic nervous system status and the treatment of cardiovascular diseases. This paper presents a mobile and real-time monitoring healthcare application of heart rate variability biofeedback, referred to as uCoherence. It consists of an automated approach to help people to voluntarily regular the autonomic system via breath control, finding the harmony point in autonomic nervous system and the best resonant frequency in cardiopulmonary system.

Keywords: heart rate variability, biofeedback, healthcare application.

1 Introduction

The autonomic nervous system (ANS) is a part of peripheral nervous system that regulates people's digestion, urination and cardiopulmonary activity. Last decades studies have witnessed the fact that many diseases are associated with the autonomic dysfunction such as asthma, cardiovascular disease (CVD), insomnia etc [1].We found that the sympathetic system (SNS), a part of ANS, always accompanies with the stress and other negative emotions, while the parasympathetic system (PSNS), the other part of ANS, can generate the happiness and other positive emotions. If people are able to voluntarily control the autonomic nerve system to reduce the sympathetic activity and increase the parasympathetic activity, they may reduce stress and anxiety, keeping their autonomic system healthy. Most autonomous functions are involuntary but a few actions can work alongside some degree of conscious control. So some efforts have been done to find the conscious control of the autonomous balance.

Heart rate variability (HRV) represents one of the most promising marker of ANS. It is a physiological phenomenon measured by the variation between the heart beat intervals [2]. The low frequency component LF (0.04 to 0.15 Hz) and the high frequency component HF (0.15 to 0.4 Hz) of HRV respectively reflect the parasympathetic and sympathetic activities [3]. Deceased PSNS activity or increased SNS activity will result in reduced HRV. It has been an emerging area that HRV measurements used in the new healthcare applications [4]. We cannot control the activity of

D. Zeng et al. (Eds.): ICSH 2013, LNCS 8040, pp. 84–95, 2013.
© Springer-Verlag Berlin Heidelberg 2013

ANS directly, but we can adjust our emotions and respiratory rhythm to improve the coherence of ANS, according to the relationship between cardiopulmonary system and ANS. In this paper we use HRV to find the autonomic balance state.

Biofeedback (BF) has been proven recently as a novel method to alter the HRV parameters and dominant rhythms in their heart activity. Miller proved that after specific biofeedback training people may learn to control the ANS with the aids of instruments [5]. The Heart Math Institute in California has promoted training in positive emotions as a basic tool for health and wellness, as a stepping stone toward optimal control of heart rate variability [6-7]. Lehrer, professor in National Institute of Health, introduce heart rate variability biofeedback in asthma therapy by examining its effects on airway reactivity and inflammation [8-9]. The current biofeedback system modalities include breathing waveform, heart rate and blood pressure [10-12].

In this paper we present a mobile, non-intrusive and real-time healthcare system, based on heart rate variability biofeedback analysis from the Electrocardiogram (ECG) and respiratory records. For each session, the system tries to find the best autonomic balance point for the trainee. It is common accepted that slow pacing breath or concentration will enhance the resonance of cardiopulmonary and increase the activity of parasympathetic nervous, which stimulate the coherence of heart and brain. In the coherence case, the amplitude of heart rate oscillations is the highest. The frequency at this point is called HRV biofeedback resonant frequency [13]. With this principle we designed and implemented an approach to find the individual resonant frequency for every trainee, then guide the trainee consciously control the heart beat to become inner peace status by audio and visual aids, which can help the trainee control the autonomic system voluntarily.

2   Methodology

2.1   System Architecture

The system architecture and all the modules of "*uCoherence*" are illustrated in Fig.1. The uCoherence consists of a uCare device, a smart phone and a server. As shown in Fig.1, there are two sensors in the uCare device: an ECG sensor and an impedance plethysmography to derive the respiratory signals. Sensors are in sensor nodes, which perform data acquisition, preprocessing and data transmission to the smart phone (or pad). The smart phone (Android based) receives data from device via Bluetooth (IEEE 802.15.1) and communicates the server through Wi-Fi (IEEE 802.11) or GPRS/3G.

The ECG data and the respiratory (RSP for short) data are processed in the smart phone by two modules: visual coherence analysis and respiratory training guidance. The coherence analysis is mainly composed of the HRV analysis and RSP analysis, as the flowchart shown in Fig.2. The visual analysis result will be treated as the feedback

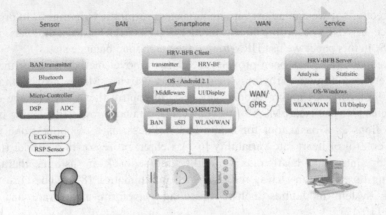

Fig. 1. System Architecture of *uCoherence*

for trainee to change the breathing speed. Both the sensor data and result will be transmitted to the server for storage and other research, which mainly contains a central database. Fig.2 illustrates the processing components of the biofeedback system, uCoherence, which will be described in the following sections.

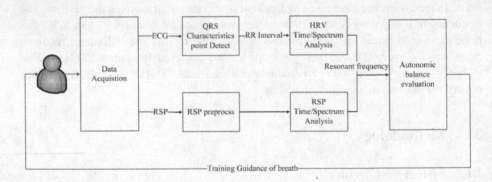

Fig. 2. Functional flow diagram of HRV biofeedback system

2.2   Signal Preprocessing

The breath training is based on the respiratory rate and the heart rate intervals. Therefore, ECG and RSP waveform is processed first to obtain the clean breath signal and the QRS complex. Both the RSP and ECG are sampled at 250 Hz in sensor nodes, which is a little bit frequent for RSP. So a down-sampling to 25Hz is done for RSP and a Butterworth filter is applied here to remove the RSP baseline drift.

The raw ECG signal is usually mixed with noise. Particularly, the main factors of the noise are baseline drifting noise caused by respiration or tiny movements of electrodes and high frequency noise imposed by electronic devices. An adaptive threshold denoising and QRS detecting method [14] based on discrete wavelet transform (DWT) is applied to achieve RR intervals. We decompose raw ECG signal in eight scales with a wavelet base function of DB4. Coefficients of scale 4 to 6 are reconstructed to restore R wave information. We seek R peak position with an adaptive threshold:

$$T = P_N + \eta(P_S - P_N)$$

(1)

Where the P_S is the running estimate of amplitude of QRS complex, P_N is running estimate of amplitude of fake QRS complex peaks and η is an adjustable coefficient. The positions of peaks of QRS complexes are marked as positions of R waves. The threshold will be updated each time an R wave is detected. Additionally, to reduce the influence of some irrational detection results, an outlier is done for the RR interval. The derived RR interval time series is denoted as $\{RR(m) : rr_i, i = 1 \cdots m\}$, where rr_i is the i th RR interval.

2.3   Autonomic Coherence Measurements

HRV Analysis

We use HRV indices as the marker of autonomic nerve system, which means the larger HRV value, the larger coherence degree. The HRV analysis is conducted by a slide window with the windows size is 256s. Principally all the HRV measurements can be used, while some are especially sensitive to biofeedback training [15]. Four time domain indices following are computed:

- standard deviation of RR interval(SDNN)
- standard deviation of differences between adjacent RR interval(SDSD)
- root mean square of successive difference(RMSSD)
- percentage of the differences between adjacent RR intervals that are greater than x milliseconds, 50 ms for example(pNNx)

We also considered the spectral analysis here. After removing of the outlier of RR interval in the preprocessing stage, the series $RR(m)$ was re-sampled at the frequency 2.0 Hz by a cubic spline interpolation. This was done because the series $RR(m)$ is un-even at the time axis. Defined X_k as the time axis:

$$X_k = \sum_{i=1}^{k} rr_i$$

(2)

For each range $[X_k, X_{k+1}]$, $k = 1 \cdots m,$ the interpolation function is constructed as follow:

$$S(x) = -\frac{(x-x_{k+1})^3}{6h_k}m_k + \frac{(x-x_k)^3}{6h_k}m_{k+1}$$

$$-(rr_k - \frac{h_k^2}{6}m_k)\frac{x-x_{k+1}}{h_k} + (rr_{k+1} - \frac{h_k^2}{6}m_{k+1})\frac{x-x_k}{h_k}$$

(3)

Where $m_k = S_k''(x_k), h_k = x_{k+1} - x_k$.

The interpolation result was illustrated in Fig.3. We can see that after the re-sampling the most glitches were removed so that the RR series was smoother.

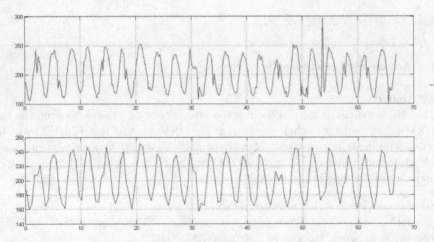

Fig. 3. RR series before and after re-sampling

Then the power spectral density (PSD) estimates using the Fast Fourier Transform (FFT) for the new even RR series. Obviously describing different ANS components function [15], four frequency domain indices are computed:

- proportion of very low frequency(pVLF)
- proportion of low frequency (pLF)
- proportion of high frequency (pHF)
- ratio of low frequency to high frequency (LF/HF)

We provide a visual real-time HRV analysis interface shown in Fig.4 for trainee to get a visual window of their ANS activity timely. We used the indices above for the respiratory training and to be the markers of the autonomic balance evaluation.

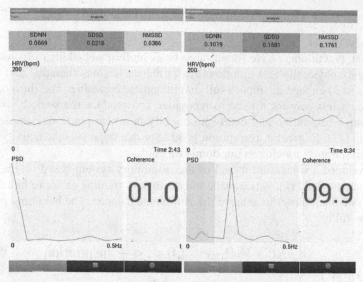

Fig. 4. HRV analysis interface: The time domain components sdnn, sdsd and rmssd were computed and update in real-time. The HRV waveform (RSA waveform) indicated the pattern state of HRV (the left one is the incoherence pattern and right one is the coherent pattern like a sinusoidal wave, which we aim to become). We also show power spectral density of HRV timely. The PSD of the coherent pattern create a spike at around 0.1 Hz.

Resonant Frequency

Current research suggests that each individual has a "resonant frequency" at which HRV is the greatest [15]. But there is no uniform "ideal value" for all persons, it is most frequently produced by persons in a fully relaxed mental state and breathing at the pace of 5~7 breaths per minute. According to Lehrer, two features [13] can be used to determine an individual's resonant frequency:

1. Paced breathing at the resonant frequency elicits the highest possible amplitude of heart rate oscillation.
2. Respiration and HRV occur in the same phase (i.e. heart rate rises simultaneously with inhalation and decreases simultaneously with exhalation)

With these two features we design an automated algorithm to find the individual's resonant frequency, and make it as the marker of autonomic balance state. As we can see in Fig.2, after the RSP and HRV analysis, we can separately get the phase of RSP φ_{rsp} and phase of HR φ_{hr}. By comparing the phase, we can used $\Delta\varphi$ to adjust the paced breathing by the feature above. $\Delta\varphi$ is defined as:

$$\Delta\varphi = \varphi_{hr} - \varphi_{rsp} \tag{4}$$

2.4   Respiratory Training Guidance and Real-Time Biofeedback

Respiratory Model

Biofeedback practitioners have found three basic biofeedback skills to increase HRV [15]: 1) relax physically and emotionally, 2) reduce anxious thoughts and negative emotions and 3) engage in smooth full diaphragmatic breathing. The third one is the fastest and easiest way for trainee to recognize and produce the smooth sinus wave form in which respiration and heart rate co-vary in a near-phase or complete phase relationship [11]. In general, respiration is a factor that depresses the activity of SNS, so we use respiratory training as our dominate guidance.

We developed a simulation model of the respiratory system based on the Warliah and Rohman method [16], which made the respiratory training closer to human physiological system and faster to achieve the autonomic balance. The breathing procedure is shown as follow:

$$V_{U_{PO}}(t) = \begin{cases} FRC + V_T(1 - e^{-2t}), 0 < t < \dfrac{T}{2}, \text{inspiration} \\ FRC + V_T(e^{T-2t} - e^{-T}), \dfrac{T}{2} < t < T, \text{exspiration} \end{cases} \tag{5}$$

The FRC is functional residual capacity in liters which is decided by the trainee's gender, age, height and weight. And the V_T means the total exchange volume in a breath.

Respiratory Training Guidance

Fig.4 shows the training guidance of our system using the model above. Based on the respiratory model, the balloon will be expanded and contracted reversely and periodically with the rhythm of the given respiratory frequency. The balloon's expansion

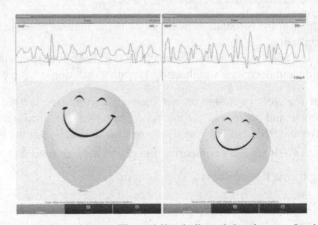

Fig. 5. Respiratory training guidance: The red line indicated the change of trainee's heart rate and the blue one indicated the respiratory. The expansion and contraction of the balloon indicated the inspiration and expiration.

indicates trainee to inhale while its contraction guides trainee to exhale. Trainee should follow the rhythm to adjust their pacing breathing. Our aim of the training here is try to make the line to be a smooth sinusoidal wave form where the heart variability is the greatest.

According to the $\Delta\varphi$ and HRV indices we can adjust the pacing breath rate using the resonant frequency feature. The rules are defined as:

$$\begin{cases} F_i = F_{i-1} + (0.5)^i, if \Delta\varphi > 0 \\ F_i = F_{i-1}, if \Delta\varphi = 0, \text{stop} \\ F_i = F_{i-1} - (0.5)^i, if \Delta\varphi < 0 \end{cases} \tag{6}$$

Where $F_0 = 10$, indicates that the respiratory rate is 6 breath per minute. Each session F_i will be last for 5 minute to be analysis. After a few sessions we can fitting out a curve of F_i and find the spike point as the resonant frequency by derivation. We use the orthogonal polynomial least square method (LSM) in the curve fitting.

We used $\Delta\varphi$ between φ_{hr} and φ_{rsp} to decide to speed up breathing or to slow down. HRV indices which we have mentioned above were used as the marker of ANS. After the fitting, we used the False Position method based on Homotopy analysis [18] to compute extreme point of the fitting function, which we consider to be the resonant frequency (RF). If $\Delta\varphi=0$, it really means that the respiratory and HRV have become coherence, where the autonomic balance reached. We also proposed a useful index Coh to score the autonomic balance. It is defined as:

$$Coh = \frac{\sum_{f=0.08}^{0.125} psd(f)}{\sum^{fs} psd(f)} \tag{7}$$

It is a useful measurement for the spike of HRV psd. The max amplitude of RR series Am_{rr} in the spectral analysis is also taken into consideration.

3   Experiment and Result

We did an experiment to validate our system. The trainee was 20 years old under the healthy condition. We took the training session with the breath rate started from 10.00 seconds per breath, then changed it to 10.25, 10.50 and 10.72 every 5 minutes, according to the adjustment rules we have talked above. After these four sessions, a fitting was done to evaluate the resonant frequency, which here we got 10.60. Then we took the final session with the respiratory rate at 10.60 seconds per breath.

The HRV analysis result was shown in Table 1. We can see that from 10.00 to 10.50, most of the HRV indices, such as SDNN, SDSD, RMSSD and pHF, were gradually increased, while in the 10.72 frequency, the values decreased. That was

Table 1. HRV analysis at difference frequency

Frsp	pNN50	SDNN	SDSD	RMSSD	pVLF	pLF	pHF	LF/HF
10.00	0.3893	0.0811	0.0326	0.0326	0.0417	0.4308	0.2148	2.0057
10.25	0.5400	0.1015	0.0378	0.0378	0.0167	0.5701	0.2851	1.9996
10.50	0.5146	0.1271	0.0483	0.0483	0.0024	0.6068	0.3562	1.7034
10.72	0.4773	0.1107	0.0364	0.0364	0.0389	0.6363	0.2624	2.4251
10.60	0.5631	0.1362	0.0522	0.0521	0.0206	0.6938	0.3540	1.9600

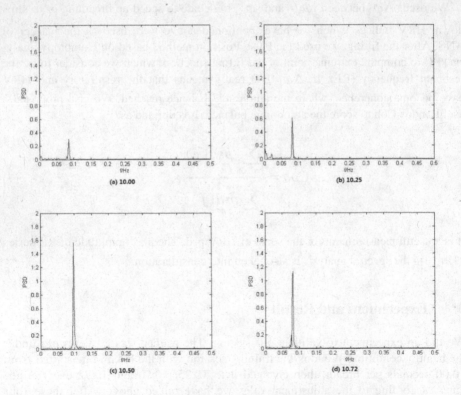

Fig. 6. PSD of different frequency from 10.00, 10.25, 10.50, 10.72

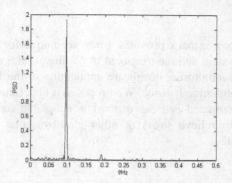

Fig. 7. PSD of the resonant frequency (10.60) evaluated from the fitting curve

because the $\Delta\varphi$ turned to negative from positive. So we can safely infer that the resonant frequency located approximately in the range of 10.50 to 10.72. At the rate of 10.60 seconds per breath we can see that the HRV indices were almost the greatest in all sessions, which strongly proved that our fitting result was nearly closed to the real resonant frequency of the subject.

The PSD, Am_{rr} and Coh also showed the same rule in our experiment, which we can see from Fig.6 to Fig.8. The peak of the PSD was increased from 10.00 to 10.50 and decreased a little at 10.72, then finally got its highest value at 10.60. The Am_{rr} and Coh index at different frequencies also showed the same trend that getting their highest value at 10.60.

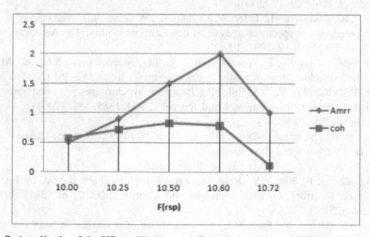

Fig. 8. Amplitude of the HR oscillation and Coherence values at different frequency

4   Conclusion

Heart rate variability biofeedback provides a new technique for the measurement of the autonomic nerve system and the treatment of cardiovascular diseases. We present a mobile and real-time monitoring healthcare application of the HRV biofeedback to help trainee to keep autonomic balance. We proposed a novel method to find the find resonant frequency automated and the method is adaptable for every trainee. The system can be used to relieve stress or other cardiovascular diseases caused by autonomic nervous system.

References

1. Wheat, A.L., Larkin, K.T.: Biofeedback of heart rate variability and related physiology: A critical review. Applied Psychophysiology and Biofeedback 35, 229–242 (2010)
2. Camm, A.J., Malik, M., Bigger, J.T., Breithardt, G., Cerutti, S., Cohen, R.J., Singer, D.H.: Heart rate variability: standards of measurement, physiological interpretation and clinical use. Task Force of the European Society of Cardiology and the North American Society of Pacing and Electrophysiology. Circulation 93, 1043–1065 (1996)
3. Acharya, U.R., Joseph, K.P., Kannathal, N., Lim, C.M., Suri, J.S.: Heart rate variability: a review. Medical and Biological Engineering and Computing 44(12), 1031–1051 (2006)
4. McCraty, R.: Heart Rhythm Coherence: An Emerging Area of Biofeedback. J. Biofeedback 30(1), 23–25 (2002)
5. Miller, N.E., Carmona, A.: Modification of a visceral response, salivation in thirsty dogs, by instrumental training with water reward. Journal of Comparative and Physiological Psychology 63(1), 1–6 (1967)
6. Childre, D., McCraty, R.: Psychophysiological correlates of spiritual experience. Biofeedback 29(4), 13–17 (2006)
7. McCraty, R., Atkinson, M., Tiller, W.A., Rein, G., Watkins, A.D.: The effects of emotions on short-term power spectrum analysis of heart rate variability. The American Journal of Cardiology 76(14), 1089–1093 (1995)
8. Lehrer, P.M., Vaschillo, E., Vaschillo, B., Lu, S.E., Scardella, A., Siddique, M., Habib, R.H.: Biofeedbacktreatment for asthma. Chest Journal 126(2), 352–361 (2004)
9. Lehrer, P., Vaschillo, E., Vaschillo, B.: Heartbeat synchronizes with respiratory rhythm only under specific circumstances. Chest Journal 126(4), 1385–1387 (2004)
10. Heart Math, CES 2013,
    http://www.heartmathstore.com/item/6400/inner-balance
11. Moss, D.: Heartratevariabilitytraining,
    http://www.bfe.org/articles/hrv.pdf
12. Zhu, Q., Zheng, F., Xie, Y.Y.: Respiratory training biofeedback system. In: International Conference Electronics, Communications and Control, ICECC, pp. 3915–3918. IEEE (September 2011)
13. Evgeny, G., Bronya, V., Paul, M.L.: Characteristics of resonance in heart rate variability stimulated by biofeedback. Applied Psychophysiology and Biofeedback 31, 129–142 (2006)
14. Li, A., Wang, S., Zhen, H., Ji, L., Wu, J.: A novel abnormal ECG beats detection method, Computer and Automation Engineering. In: The 2nd International Conference, ICCAE, pp. 47–51 (2010)

15. Moss, D.: Heart rate variability and biofeedback. Psychophysiology Today: The Magazine for Mind-Body Medicine 1, 4–11 (2004)
16. Warliah, L., Rohman, A.S., Rusmin, P.H.: Model Development of Air Volume and Breathing Frequency in Human Respiratory System Simulation. Procedia-Social and Behavioral Sciences 67, 260–268 (2012)
17. Lehrer, P.M., Vaschillo, E., Vaschillo, B.: Resonant frequency biofeedback training to increase cardiac variability: Rationale and manual for training. Applied Psychophysiology and Biofeedback 25(3), 177–191 (2000)
18. Abbasbandy, S.: A new modification of false position method based on homotopy analysis method. Applied Mathematics and Mechanics 29(2), 223–228 (2008)

Bootstrapping Activity Modeling
for Ambient Assisted Living

Jie Wan, Michael J. O'Grady, and Gregory M.P. O'Hare

CLARITY Centre for Sensor Web Technologies,
University College Dublin, Ireland
jie.wan@ucdconnect.ie, {michael.ogrady,gregory.ohare}@ucd.ie

Abstract. In many societies, the age profile of the population is increasing, posing many challenges for societies, health services and carers. One response to this unfolding situation has been to direct research effort towards Ambient Assisted Living (AAL), specifically, its enabling technologies. A critical impediment to the deployment of such systems remains the accurate and timely identification of the Activities of Daily Living (ADLs). This paper advocates a minimalist approach to ADL recognition; rather than capturing all possible ADLs, the reliable identification of a select subset of ADLs may prove sufficient for many categories of AAL services. A methodology is described and initial results presented.

Keywords: Ambient Assisted Living, Activity Recognition, User Modeling.

1   Introduction

Global Aging is a success story and is testimony to medical and public health advances that have occurred in recent decades. Yet this success will invariably incur a cost over time. By 2025, one in five Europeans will be more than 65 years old, up from 16% in 2002. The percentage of those active in the workforce will shrink or decrease, while an increasing elderly population will have to be supported. In line with this increasing aging profile is a projected increase in the incidence of dementia, especially Alzheimer's Disease (AD). It is estimated that there were over 35 million people with AD in 2010, and this is projected to increase to 65.7 million by 2030 [1]. While this is essentially a societal problem, Ambient Assisted Living (AAL) [10] has been proposed as a technological solution for those whose independence is potentially compromised either though old age or ill-health.

Fundamental to many categories of AAL is a user or behaviour model. Using such a model as a base line, opportunities for assistance may be identified. Furthermore, longitudinal monitoring and analysis may be undertaken. One aspect of AAL concerns Activities of Daily Living (ADLs). Recognizing these is essential as it enables deviations from normal behaviour be identified thus providing insights into possible illnesses, deteriorating health or the identification of potentially life-threatening situations. While the variety of ADLs is large, it may be hypothesized that within the

D. Zeng et al. (Eds.): ICSH 2013, LNCS 8040, pp. 96–106, 2013.

home, at least initially, there is a certain set of activities that are performed on a regular basis and are shared across populations. In identifying this subset, it may be envisaged that AAL deployments may function quicker and more robustly than would otherwise be the case. Furthermore, the possibility of a behaviour model becoming applicable to a broader population, rather than just the individual, may arise. In this way, such a general model could prove a basis for rapidly constructing models that would be more personalized to the individual and their situation. This paper seeks to demonstrate the viability of such an approach to user model construction for AAL scenarios.

This paper is structured as follows: Section 2 presents pertinent related research in technologies cognizant to AAL. A prototypical AAL configuration is outlined in Section 3. The methodology engaged for activity recognition, and initial results, are presented in Section 4. Section 5 outlines some ongoing research after which the paper is concluded.

2   Related Research

Human activity recognition offers extraordinary opportunities for Ambient Assisted Living (AAL); it is fundamental to one of the critical characteristics of AAL, that of being capable of understanding the behavior, routines and needs of older adults, as well as evolving to meet their needs as circumstances change [5]. The idea of adopting sensors and sensor networks for activity monitoring and recognition has been prevalent for a couple of decades. A large range of sensors have been manufactured and deployed to enable smart monitoring. A number of smart home projects have been documented, for example, MavHome [3], the GatorTech Smart House [4].

Research in activity recognition has been extensive; various activity recognition systems and techniques have been developed. For example, [14] describes a system that recognizes activities in the home, utilizing a set of simple and ubiquitous sensors. Manual activity annotation method is implemented using a PDA device. [18] presents a multi-model system that aims at recognizing multiuser activities within a sensor network embedded smart home. The target users are assigned a set of wearable sensors. In addition, [8] presents a prototype that extract and label a person's activities and significant places from the traces of GPS data, utilizing the Relational Markov Network (RMN) Model.

On the other hand, in the outdoor scenario, GPS has prevalent for years. Numerous tracking & navigation systems for the elderly, children and pets have been developed, such as [12]. Moreover, the smart-phone has become central to mobile computing, as it offers richer functionalities enabled by a growing number of inbuilt sensors. Countless smart phone based healthcare applications have been developed, examples includes [13], [7].

Research in pervasive healthcare has gained significant success, as numerous aspects have been investigated extensively. However, there is an urgent need for an integrated service, which is capable of monitoring and tracking users both indoor and

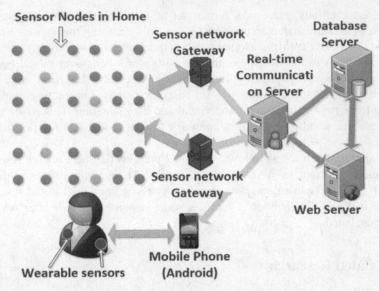

Fig. 1. Architecture AAL System

outdoor, correctly and accurately recognizing users' behavior, and identifying certain deviations to avoid the occurrence of risky situations. Fundamental to the adoption of such systems is a sophisticated behaviour modeling methodology for ADL recognition that minimizes the time required for learning user preferences.

3   Holistic Solution

An initial prototype has been implemented; this was extended from previous research [16]. It includes several functioning components:

— Monitoring. The monitoring component is fabricated based upon a typical AAL configuration, which is a rich sensor-embedded smart home, as well as a GPS enabled mobile phone system that facilitates tracking & positioning in an outdoor scenario.

— Sensor Data Collection. Sensor data is transmitted to a central station for further processing. To facilitate the heterogeneity of the sensor network, a middleware solution [11] is employed. An Android smart phone serves both as a sensor gateway, which transmits sensor data to the server, and as a GPS position provider.

— Activity Recognition and Pattern Analysis. Sensor data is utilized for situation and behavior recognition, harnessing a variety of machine-learning techniques.

— Web Services, which offers a remote interface, especially for associated carers and stakeholders, so as to obtain information in real time.

The system architecture is demonstrated in Figure. 1.

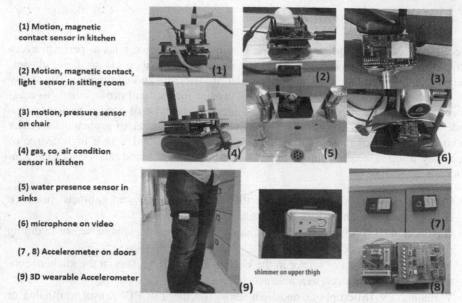

(1) Motion, magnetic contact sensor in kitchen

(2) Motion, magnetic contact, light sensor in sitting room

(3) motion, pressure sensor on chair

(4) gas, co, air condition sensor in kitchen

(5) water presence sensor in sinks

(6) microphone on video

(7 , 8) Accelerometer on doors

(9) 3D wearable Accelerometer

Fig. 2. Samples of Sensor Installation in the Smart Home

3.1 Sensor Embedded Smart Home

Sensors are the fundamental elements for enabling smart environments, offering an extraordinary basis for the delivery of AAL services. Instead of mounting a large number of wearable sensors on the human body, a set of sensors are identified and installed within the smart home. Numerous categories of sensors are have been harnessed:

— Contact sensors are deployed to sense any interaction with specified objects.
— Motion sensors, of the PIR variety, detect the presence and movement of any object or person. Motion sensors are distributed in various locations, approximately every four meters given their sensing range.
— Accelerometers, with X-Y-Z axes are attached onto doors and other specified objects, to sense movement. In addition, wearable accelerometers that are used to measure the movements of walking, sitting, and standing.
— Pressure sensors are installed on chairs for the detection of sitting and rising.
— Ambient environmental sensors are configured to monitor temperature, humidity, light and background noise.
— Water presence sensors, which are installed in the baths, showers and sinks, indicate certain behaviors according to their location.
— Gas sensors complete the configuration of smart home; these can detect the emission of gas and smoke, but have been included from a safety perspective rather than that of recognizing ADLs.
— GPS empowers the outdoor localization; it is shipped with the Android smart phone.

Fig.2 exemplifies a few samples of the deployed sensors in the smart home.

4   Activity Recognition

Recall ADLs are defined as the routine activities that people tend to perform every day without needing assistance. ADLs are generally described via six basic classes, namely, eating, bathing, dressing, using toilet, transferring and continence. The ability of a dependent person to perform ADLs is crucial for medical professionals to diagnose possible latent health conditions and identify the type of caring service to provide if required. Based upon the above definition, a number of archetypical ADLs have been identified that could, it is envisaged, be identified with a high degree of accuracy using a sensor configuration. A number of ADLs and their associated sensors are as follows:

— Cooking (Contact sensors on the kettle, tea, coffee and cup cabinets, presence (PIR) sensor in kitchen, wearable accelerometer)
— Having a meal (Pressure mat on the chairs, PIR, light, microphone sensor in dining room, wearable accelerometer)
— Washing dishes (Water sensor in the kitchen sink, PIR sensors in the kitchen, contact sensors on cabinets, wearable accelerometer)
— Watching TV (Microphone and light sensor on the TV, PIR sensor in dinning or bed rooms, pressure mat on chairs, wearable accelerometer)
— Using toilet (PIR sensor in toilet, wearable accelerometer)
— Washing hands (PIR, water sensor in sink, wearable accelerometer)
— Go to bed / Get up (Pressure mat near the bed, various sensors in bed room and other rooms)
— Going out / Coming home (Contact sensor on the front door, GPS signal status)
— Going to Church (GPS, geographic, Zones,)
— Shopping (GPS, geographic, Zones)
— Go to Restaurant (GPS, geographic, Zones)
— Meeting Friends (GPS, geographic, Zones)

The outdoor component is extended from WanderHelp, and a detailed description of the architecture may be found elsewhere [15] [16]. The outdoor service is implemented as a map based tracking system, allowing the definition of zones and personalized alarm-raising protocols. Moreover, it communicates with both the elderly user and their carer in an as-needed basis. The decision capability concerning user's behavior as it relates to zone intrusion is enabled by the WanderHelp service, an example of web interface is depicted in Fig. 3. Zones are defined according to individual user's daily routine, to partition outdoor environment in both the spatial and temporal dimensions. Three types of zones are included that are the green, red and amber. Green zones defines the areas that are assumed to be safe all the times, which is usually immediately adjacent to the home. Red zones indicate the areas that are considered to be dangerous to elderly users, in case of wandering, a railway station is an obvious examples. Amber zones are dynamic and dependent upon the temporal dimension, which specifies the areas where users are allowed to visit at certain time only.

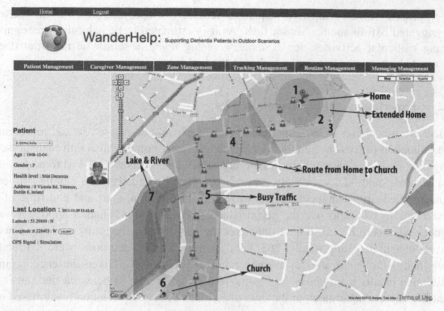

Fig. 3. An example of Web Interface for Outdoor Tracking System

4.1   Activity Recognition Methodology

Given the fact that sensor data is usually noisy and ambiguous, learning based proba-bilistic algorithms (Bayesian Theory, J48) are applied with a set of temporal features [17]. Firstly, the time series are divided into time intervals with a constant length, named Δt, the value of sensor i is represented by x_t^i, which indicates whether sensor i is fired at least once during time t to $t + \Delta t$. Additionally, we bring another temporal feature, that is, the time latency, named x_l^i, which specifies how long has sensor i been fired for the given activity. Hence, s denotes the number of sensors that are deployed, then the sensor observation at time t can be defined as $X_t = \{(x_t^1, x_l^1), (x_t^2, x_l^2) ...(x_t^s, x_l^s)\}$. Given user annotated activity label at, which symbolizes the activity at time t. $q_t \in A = \{a_1, a_2, a_3, ...a_n\}$, where n indicated the number of ADLs that are labeled. Consequently, utilizing the above-mentioned algorithms, the activity recognition model can be constructed as $f(x) = P(A|X)$ that is the probabilistic distribution of the activity labels given the sensor reading, which can be utilized to predict the corresponding label for a new instance of feature X. Moreover, to achieve a better performance, three approaches are adopted to examine such learning algorithms:

- Approach - A, time intervals Δt is set as 60 seconds, whilst absolute time is adopted to classify the ADLs.
- Approach - B, in this approach, a temporal feature is added, where time series are clustered into 7 categories, which are early *morning, morning, noon, early after-noon, late afternoon, early evening, late evening* and *night*. As some activities may only occur in certain time, for example, having breakfast may only take place in the morning.

— Approach - C, an additional sequential feature is employed, which is the sensor triggered before another sensor fires. As it is estimated to be helpful for recognizing particular activities, for example, *comeing home*, a sensor on the front door would be triggered before the sensor in the hall fires.

4.2   Experiment and Evaluation Results

There are two phases of the experiment, named $phase^1$ and $phase^2$. $Phase^1$ represents the validation process in a laboratory simulated smart home whilst with realistic setting. During $phase^1$, a number of randomly selected subjects were asked to perform a list of predefined ADLs. Activity data was annotated manually via a mobile application installed on a handheld device, to record the location, start and end time of a given activity. To appraise the performance, K-fold cross validation approach was conducted, where K = 10, Fig. 4 illustrates the classification result by applying Naïve bayes classifier. With totally 263 valid activities, 228 activities were correctly classified, which indicates an average accuracy of 88.46%. Given the encouraging validation results from $phase^1$ and to move forward, $phase^2$ is being carried out in a real life one-bed apartment, at the time of writing. To date, evaluation result based on initial one-month experiment in $phase^2$ has been obtained.

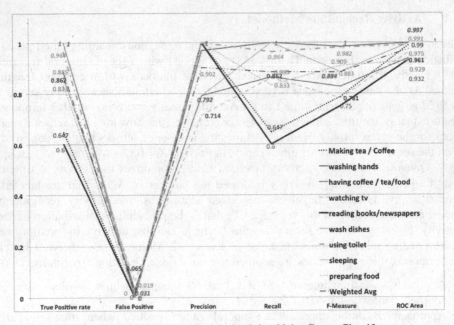

Fig. 4. Initial Validation Result Applying Naive Bayes Classifer

Table 1. Evaluation Results for all Classified Activities Applying J48 Classifier

J48 Classifier	Approach - A	Approach - B	Approach - C
Average Weighted Accuracy	90.38%	90.38%	92.35%
Average Weighted Precision	89.63%	89.64%	91.67%
Average Weighted True Positive	90.38%	90.38%	92.35%
Average Weighted FMeasure	88.78%	88.78%	91.31%

Table 2. Evaluation Results for all Classified Activities Applying Naive Bayes Classifier

Naive Bayes Classifier	Approach - A	Approach - B	Approach - C
Average Weighted Accuracy	83.98%	83.98%	83.47%
Average Weighted Precision	82.81%	82.81%	83.21%
Average Weighted True Positive	83.98%	83.98%	83.47%
Average Weighted FMeasure	82.62%	82.62%	82.49%

Provided the annotated dataset in *phase*², the leave one day out validation approach is performed, where Table.1 illustrates the classification results of applying J48 classifier utilizing the above-mentioned approaches. Meanwhile, Table.2 indicates the validation results of adopting Naive Bayes Classifier. As is depicted, J48 points out a better results consistent with a number of evaluation criteria. On the other hand, in comparison with *Approach - A*, no significant improvement is gained by *Approach - B*. Whilst *Approach - C* indicates a better performance on certain activities.

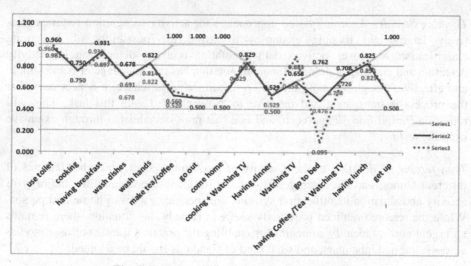

Fig. 5. Experiment Result Applying J48 Classifier

Fig. 5 demonstrates the classification results of a number of ADLs, applying the J48 classifier, where *series 3* depicts the classification results utilizing *Approach - C*, while *series 2* presents the classification results using *Approach - B*, in addition to *series 1* presents the results of *Approach - A*. As is demonstrated, no significant difference is presented between *series 2* and *series 1*. Moreover, *series 3* presents substantial improvement on several activities; such as *come home, go out, go to bed* and *get up*. Nonetheless, a number of other characteristics may have meaningful impact on the validation results, for example, the structure and deployment of the sensor network, the location of the sensor nodes, the errors and missing values in the recording of the ground truth, especially when manual annotation method is adopted, as well as the specification of activity boundaries. Such issues will be discovered and evaluated in the future. Furthermore, human behaviour tends to be more complicated and diverse in practice than performing predefined activities in the laboratory, for example, multiple activities may be overlapped or interconnected, such as watching TV and having a meal. Thus, in the system, several combinations of such activities are highlighted and classified as a single separate activity, for an instance, *cooking + watching TV, having meal + watching TV*.

5   Ongoing Research

As was discussed, the *phase*^{2} experiment are currently ongoing with the objective of developing a more generic user model. In addition, a number of other aspects are currently under investigation.

Training Samples. Learning based approaches for activity recognition requires relatively large valid training examples to avoid the possibility of inaccurate classification. Moreover, activity data annotation is a key determinant of activity detection and classifier training. Manual annotation has the advantage of being simple and effective, though it is not perfect. To maximize performance, it is necessary that the process is transparent and intuitive to those charged with this task. This will require a *Design For All* approach, and one that must be validated through extensive usability testing.

Transferable Model. Due to the diversity of the layouts, sizes, and other features of different homes, and the heterogeneity of the inhabitant population, the majority of activity and situation identification systems are specific to a given home and person. While the research outlined previously seeks to remedy this situation, there remains an urgent need to identify strategies for enabling the practical transfer of user models across home and inhabitant, and what kind of standards should be adopted.

Online Real-time Activity Recognition. There is an urgent need that users' behavior information can be obtained by the authorized carers and stakeholders remotely in real time. Thus a more scalable and robust user model is requisite, one that is capable of recognizing user behavior, and deviations thereof, based on streaming sensor data. Web services are being considered as a means of enabling such functionality.

Interpreting and Collaborating with Other Smart Home Datasets. As of now, many smart home-based human activity datasets are available publicly, such as the *Placelab* data provided by MIT [9], *CASAS* dataset collected by Washington State University (WSU) [2], and *CodeFramework* from Intelligent System Lab Amsterdam [6]. Having validated the approach in a real home, it is intended to harness these datasets for further validation of the various activity-recognition algorithms.

Decoupling the Sensor Infrastructure. Currently, ADLs and their enabling behavior models are tightly coupled to a particular sensing infrastructure. A prerequisite for more robust and scalable models is to decouple the sensing infrastructure. This raises issues of a standardization and ontological nature. It is intended to investigate how more abstract models of sensing components could be adopted to enable the adoption of a broader category and combination of physical sensor.

6   Conclusion

A key challenge in AAL is to minimize the time span between an AAL configuration being physically deployed, and it proceeding to function as expected and to the user's requirements. One key reason for this time lapse is due to the time required for the AAL system to learn the routines and behaviours of the person in question. This paper described an approach to minimize this time lapse through the harnessing of generic ADLs as a means of seeding the initial user models necessary for the AAL configuration to commence operating in the expected manner.

Acknowledgment. This work is supported by Science Foundation Ireland (SFI) under grant 07/CE/I1147.

References

1. Alzheimer's Disease International. World Alzheimer report (2012)
2. Cook, D., Krishnan, N., Rashidi, P.: Activity discovery and activity recognition: A new partnership. IEEE Transactions on Cybernetics 43(3), 820–828 (2013)
3. Cook, D., Youngblood, M., Heierman, I., Gopalratnam, E.O.K., Rao, S., Litvin, A., Khawaja, F.: Mavhome: an agent-based smart home. In: Proceedings of the First IEEE International Conference on Pervasive Computing and Communications (PerCom 2003), pp. 521–524 (2003)
4. Helal, S., Mann, W., El-Zabadani, H., King, J., Kaddoura, Y., Jansen, E.: The GatorTech smart house: a programmable pervasive space. Computer 38(3), 50–60 (2005)
5. Hu, D.H., Zheng, V.W., Yang, Q.: Cross-domain activity recognition via transfer learning. Pervasive and Mobile Computing 7(3), 344–358 (2011)
6. Kersten, M.L., Manegold, S., Mullender, K.S.: The database architectures research group at CWI. ACM SIGMOD Record 40(4), 39–44 (2011)

7. Kwapisz, J.R., Weiss, G.M., Moore, S.A.: Activity recognition using cell phone accel-erometers. SIGKDD Explor. Newsl. 12(2), 74–82 (2011)
8. Liao, L., Patterson, D.J., Fox, D., Kautz, H.: Learning and inferring transportation routines. Artificial Intelligence 171, 311–331 (2007)
9. Logan, B., Healey, J., Philipose, M., Tapia, E.M., Intille, S.S.: A long-term evaluation of sensing modalities for activity recognition. In: Krumm, J., Abowd, G.D., Seneviratne, A., Strang, T. (eds.) UbiComp 2007. LNCS, vol. 4717, pp. 483–500. Springer, Heidelberg (2007)
10. O'Hare, G.M.P., Muldoon, C., O'Grady, M.J., Collier, R.W., Mupdoch, O., Carr, D.: Sensor web interaction. International Journal on Artificial Intelligence Tools 21(02), 1240006 (2012)
11. O'Grady, M.J., Muldoon, C., Dragone, M., Tynan, R., O'Hare, G.M.P.: Towards evolutio-nary ambient assisted living systems. Journal of Ambient Intelligence and Humanized Computing 1(1), 15–29 (2010)
12. Paiva, S., Abreu, C.: Low cost GPS tracking for the elderly and Alzheimer patients. Procedia Technology 5, 793–802 (2012)
13. Pigadas, V., Doukas, C., Plagianakos, V.P., Maglogiannis, I.: Enabling constant moni-toring of chronic patient using android smart phones. In: 4th International Conference on Pervasive Technologies Related to Assistive Environments, pp. 63:1–63:2. ACM (2011)
14. Tapia, E.M., Intille, S.S., Larson, K.: Activity recognition in the home using simple and ubiquitous sensors. In: Ferscha, A., Mattern, F. (eds.) PERVASIVE 2004. LNCS, vol. 3001, pp. 158–175. Springer, Heidelberg (2004)
15. Wan, J., Byrne, C., O'Hare, G.M.P., O'Grady, M.J.: OutCare: Supporting Dementia Patients in Outdoor Scenarios. In: Setchi, R., Jordanov, I., Howlett, R.J., Jain, L.C. (eds.) KES 2010, Part IV. LNCS, vol. 6279, pp. 365–374. Springer, Heidelberg (2010)
16. Wan, J., O'Grady, M.J., O'Hare, G.M.: Towards Cross Senseor Network Activity Rec-ognition for Ambient Assisted Living. In: 7th Annual Irish HCI Conference, Dundalk, Ireland. ACM (June 2013)
17. Wang, L., Gu, T., Tao, X., Chen, H., Lu, J.: Recognizing multi-user activities using wear-able sensors in a smart home. Pervasive Mob. Comput. 7, 287–298 (2011)

Healthcare Information System: A Facilitator of Primary Care for Underprivileged Elderly via Mobile Clinic

Kup-Sze Choi, Rebecca K.P. Wai, and Esther Y.T. Kwok

Centre for Integrative Digital Health, School of Nursing
The Hong Kong Polytechnic University
{thomasks.choi,rebecca.wai,yeung.tsz.kwok}@polyu.edu.hk

Abstract. Ageing is a global challenge. As health conditions gradually deteriorate, elders are prone to suffering from multiple chronic diseases. The impact of ageing on the heath system is therefore unprecedented. Primary and preventive care is important to ensure older adults to receive immediate healthcare so that their health problems can be handled and alleviated in a timely manner, thus reducing the risk of development into serious illnesses. However, degradation of mobility in elderly becomes a hurdle to the access of healthcare services. In the paper, we present an outreach community healthcare model via a mobile clinic, which provides health assessment, interventions and health education to community-dwelling elderly. A key highlight of the mobile healthcare model is the adoption of healthcare information system (HIS) to streamline the operations and to enable smooth service delivery even with tight human resource. The role of information technology, the resulting benefits and outcomes are discussed in the paper. The HIS-leveraged mobile healthcare model is highly praised by the community and serves as an exemplar for establishing mobile clinics for various healthcare services.

Keywords: Healthcare information system, primary care, preventive care, telehealth, mobile clinic, ageing, elderly.

1   Introduction

Ageing population is a global issue. According to the World Health Organization, 1.2 billion people in the world will reach the age of 60 or above in 2025 [1]. As pointed out by the Department of Economic and Social Affairs of the United Nations, population ageing is unprecedented, pervasive and enduring [2]. Considerable increase in the demand of healthcare and long-term care is becoming a major challenge to the society. Here, primary and preventive care is important to ensure older adults to access appropriate health assessment, receive timely health treatment, and also to equip them with health literacy, by which their health problems can be handled and alleviated in a timely manner so that the risk of development into serious illnesses can be reduced. However, degradation of mobility in older adults becomes a hurdle to the access of healthcare services, particularly for community-dwelling elderly who cannot afford

D. Zeng et al. (Eds.): ICSH 2013, LNCS 8040, pp. 107–112, 2013.

the medical expenses and transportation cost. As a result, they may neglect their health problems and miss the best opportunities for early treatment, thereby placing immense pressure on secondary and tertiary care.

In the regard, we advocate outreach healthcare model to deliver primary and preventive care services to needy older adults. The services are provided on vehicle that serves a mobile clinic for health assessment, intervention, health education and promotion. A key highlight of mobile healthcare model is the adoption of healthcare information system (HIS) to streamline the operations and to enable smooth service delivery even with tight human resource. Following a brief description of the background and services the outreach mobile clinic, the paper focuses on the infrastructure, system framework and features of the information systems developed to facilitate health services delivery.

2   Outreach Mobile Healthcare Model

The outreach mobile healthcare model is implemented in Hong Kong, with a population of 7 million people where approximately 12% aged 65 or above. In line with the global trend, the figure is projected to 26% in 2036 [3]. Furthermore, 75% of the people in this age group are suffering from one or more chronic diseases [4]. To meet the resulting challenge to the healthcare system, the outreach healthcare model is realized with a mobile clinic, where an integrative approach is adopted for delivering primary and preventive care services to needy older adults. On a vehicle commuting to public housing estates on daily basis, the mobile clinic offers free health services to community-dwelling elderly aged 60 or above, administered by a team of advanced practice nurses (APNs). The services include basic bio-measurements as well as assessment of cognition, mood, pain, nutrition, mobility, visual acuity, oral hygiene and constipation. Health education, programmes on the management of pain or constipation, workshops on hypertension and counseling services are also provided as necessary. Referrals to mainstream health services are made for cases requiring immediate medical treatments. The model is proven to be an effective way to promote good health for older adults, where their health conditions are monitored to enable early detection and treatment and prevent reoccurrence. Education is also provided to improve health literacy, thereby empowering the elderly to become responsible for their own health. In addition to providing healthcare services, the mobile clinic is also used as a platform for nursing student placement and health research.

3   The Healthcare Information System

3.1   Needs Assessment

The service capacity of the mobile clinic is to provide healthcare to 1,500 individual clients with a total of 8,000 visits per year. The duration of each visit is 45 minutes. The workflow of the services is as follows. First, clients are registered to create a new account or retrieve their health history. *Preliminary health assessments* are then performed, e.g. bio-measurements and happiness test. Depending on the initial results, appropriate *focus assessments* are conducted by APNs to carry out in-depth investigation about the health problems. These include assessment of nutrition level, cognitive status, mobility, or pain and physical conditions. Interventions and follow-up treatments are then provided accordingly. On occasions where the problems persist or immediate medical follow-up are required, referrals are made by the APNs of the mobile clinic. The workflow is illustrated in Fig. 1.

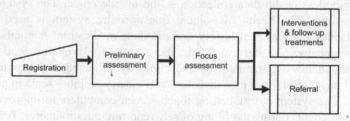

Fig. 1. Basic workflow of the mobile clinic

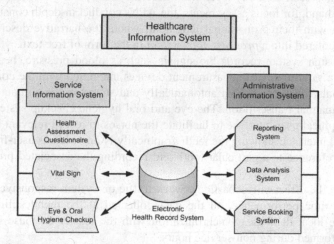

Fig. 2. Framework of the healthcare information system of the mobile clinic

3.2   System Framework

The HIS is designed to meet the needs of the mobile clinic and the workflow. Regarding the infrastructure for information exchange, a local area network is set up at the mobile clinic, where a local database server is installed for storing the data recorded with the computers in the clinic. As the healthcare services are provided on a mobile vehicle, communication with the main office is established through internet access via 3G network or Wi-Fi, depending on network availability at service locations. Nurses at the mobile clinic can remotely access the information systems and the master database, i.e. the electronic health record system, back in the main office. The data are encrypted before transmission over the network. The HIS developed for the mobile clinic consists of two main parts, namely, the *service information system* and the *administrative information system*, as shown Fig. 2. The systems are all web-based, implemented on the Microsoft Windows platform. The databases are designed with the relational approach using Microsoft SQL. The HL7 Clinical Document Architecture is adopted to model the health data collected in the mobile clinic [5].

Service Information System. The primary role of the service information system is to enable paperless health data collection at the mobile clinic. The system contains three subsystems. The health assessment questionnaire system is used to record client's personal data, medical history and previous medication. A number of electronic questionnaires are integrated into the system for preliminary assessments. These questionnaires are standardized and clinically validated, e.g. happiness scale, abbreviated mental test, brief pain inventory and elderly mobility scale in preliminary assessment. The system is installed on touch screen computers to improve usability and to engage clients during the filling of self-reporting questionnaires. For example, the pain assessment questionnaire is presented with graphics to allow clients to directly point at the screen the body locations where they feel painful, as shown in Fig. 3. On the other hand, for focus assessments, the APNs conduct in-depth consultation and investigation with their professional judgment, where the narrative descriptions and findings are entered into a *progress note system* in the form of free text.

The vital sign system records bio-signals such as blood pressure, heart rate and blood oxygen saturation with measurement devices integrated with the computers, so that the signals can be measured automatically and stored in the computers without the need of manual transcription. The eye and oral hygiene checkup system provides intuitive graphical user interface to facilitate the nurses to record relevant health data. In particular, interface showing the teeth graphically is provided as user-friendly way for making reference to a particular tooth and recording the associated problems (see Fig. 3).

To reduce the effect of stochastic network traffic on system responsiveness and to achieve real-time performance, all the data collected at the mobile clinic are first stored in the local database. Synchronization with the master database in the main office is performed during non-service hours.

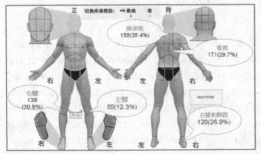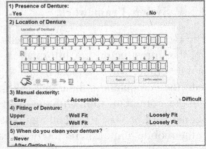

Fig. 3. Screenshots of the pain assessment (left) and the oral hygiene checkup system (right)

Administrative Information System. The administrative information system is developed to improve the service efficiency and to reduce administrative workload of the nurses. The service booking system is a critical component that is used to schedule and manage clients' appointments, registering the services to be offered and the responsible nurses. An administrative assistant is employed to make telephone booking with the clients according to the timing for next visit as specified the nurses based on the health screening results. The assistant also refers to the booking system to make reminder calls to the elderly for upcoming visits. Screenshots of the system are shown in Fig. 4.

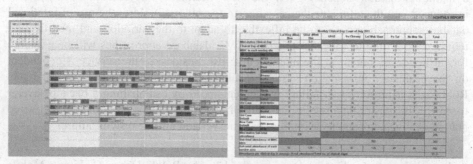

Fig. 4. Screenshots of the booking system: daily schedule (left), monthly summary (right)

Refer to Fig. 2, the reporting system is used to query the data stored in the electronic health record systems for the generation of monthly and annual reports on the service volume (e.g. frequency of visits and services provided) as well as statistics concerning demographics, health problems and referrals. Detailed search and analysis of information in the electronic health record system can also be performed with the data analysis system, where a text search engine is provided for fast and accurate data retrieval. Query of a specific vital sign or a particular item in the electronic questionnaires can be made with the system. In particular, the text search engine also provides a convenient way to retrieve data from the free-text narration of the focus assessments for qualitative research.

4   Discussion and Conclusion

This paper presents the actual implementation of the outreach healthcare model with a mobile vehicle. The mobile clinic was established in 2008 for underprivileged elderly. On average, the clinic serves around 6,000 client visits annually. Besides, about 200 referrals are made per year for health problems identified that require further medical treatments. Post-referral follow up has shown that the corresponding medical decisions are in line with the results of health assessments conducted at the mobile clinic, which indicates the significance of the outreach healthcare model in preventive and primary care. Over the five years of service, the mobile clinic has been accepted and proven to be a viable and effective primary care model by the community, and established itself as an exemplar of outreach healthcare. The proposed model is also adopted for the provision of other mobile healthcare services, e.g. dementia care.

A success factor for smooth implementation of the mobile clinic is the healthcare information system. The system enables reliable health data management as well as timely and accurate information retrieval, making it possible to delivery healthcare service with minimal human resource. The information system also facilitates the acquisition of service data for effective management of the clinic's operations, and also streamlines the mining of necessary data for reviewing clients' health conditions.

Like other medical data, the information associated with the mobile clinic is also dynamic in nature, depending on the new healthcare services and assessments introduced into the clinic, or the cessation of the old ones. Here, the use of relational database approach appears to be inflexible to adapt to the variation and modification required from time to time. To this end, XML database approaches will be explored for further development of the mobile clinic [6]. Besides, as the service is dependent on the healthcare information system, availability of the system is a critical issue. Robustness against system failure will be enhanced by establishing a backup severer to mirror the master database in the main office, so that the service can be recovered automatically and promptly with minimal intervention during system failure.

Acknowledgements. The work is supported by the PolyU-Henry G. Leong Mobile Integrative Health Centre which is funded by a generous donation from the Tai Hung Fai Charity Foundation established by the philanthropist Dr. Edwin S.H. Leong.

References

1. Elder maltreatment. Media Center. World Health Organization, http://www.who.int/mediacentre/factsheets/fs357/en/
2. World Population Ageing: 1950-2050. Department of Economic and Social Affairs, Population Division. United Nation, http://www.un.org/esa/population/publications/worldageing19502050/
3. The Ageing Trend of the Hong Kong Population Continues. Census and Statistics Department, The Hong Kong Special Administrative Region, China, http://www.censtatd.gov.hk/FileManager/EN/Content_1064/B1_E.pdf
4. Report on Healthy Ageing Executive Summary. Elderly Commission, The Hong Kong Special Administrative Region, China, http://www.elderlycommission.gov.hk/en/library/Ex-sum.htm
5. Dolin, R.H., Alschuler, L., Boyer, S., Beebe, C., Behlen, F.M., Biron, P.V., Shvo, A.S.: HL7 Clinical Document Architecture, Release 2. Journal of American Medical Informatics Association 13, 30–39 (2006)
6. Lee, K.Y., Tang, W.C., Choi, K.S.: Alternatives to Relational Database: Comparison of NoSQL and XML Approaches for Clinical Data Storage. Computer Methods and Programs in Biomedicine 110, 99–109 (2013)

Kalico: A Smartphone Application
for Health-Smart Menu Selection within a Budget

Mohd Anwar[1,*], Edward Hill[1], John Skujins[1], Kitty Huynh[2], and Cristopher Doss[2]

[1] Dept. of Computer Science, North Carolina A&T State University
Greensboro, NC, USA
[2] Dept. of Computer Engineering, North Carolina A&T State University
Greensboro, NC, USA
{manwar,cdoss}@ncat.edu

Abstract. Smartphone apps are increasingly in use for personalized and preventive health and wellness management. Many preventive and manageable health conditions such as obesity, diabetes, and hypertension can be addressed through proper smartphone-based dietary interventions. Our research aims at developing a smartphone-based dietary software that helps users select a healthy eat-out menu item within a budget. To this end, our contribution in this research is three-fold: first, we identify gaps in existing smartphone apps; second, we elicit requirements for a smartphone-based dietary intervention app; third, following the elicited requirements, we design and develop an android app.

Keywords: smartphone, personalized health, android app, dietary interventions.

1 Introduction

The popularlity of smartphones and tablets (e.g., nearly half (46%) of American adults are smartphone owners as of February 2012[1]) is the key factor in the increasing growth of mobile health technology. Smartphones offer ubiquity and pervasiveness, making it a point-of-need personal essential. While mobile communication facility is the primary purpose of a smartphone, it offers an enormous opportunity for wellness promotion and wellbeing management.

Smartphone is the best means to reach out to wider population. Mobile subscribers are expected to reach 6.9 billion by the end of 2013[2]. As a result, the mobile health research community is poised to take full advantage of smartphone technology. The powerful computing capability, capacious memories, and open operating systems of smartphones encourage application development. Lane et al. [2] observes that the rapid growth of smartphone health apps is driven by (i) near-zero user effort and (ii) universal access by means of just a single download from the smartphone app repository.

---

* Corresponding author.
[1] http://pewinternet.org/Reports/2012/Smartphone-Update-2012.aspx
[2] http://www.portioresearch.com/media/1797/Mobile%20Factbook%202012.pdf

D. Zeng et al. (Eds.): ICSH 2013, LNCS 8040, pp. 113–121, 2013.
© Springer-Verlag Berlin Heidelberg 2013

Our focus in this research is how to promote healhy dietary habits. In our fast-paced life, a significant portion of our food consumptions take place in restaurants and eateries. Food from fast-food and casual dining restaurants are generally higher in calories and less healthy than foods prepared at home [19]. A study [19] further suggests that when dining out, people eat more food, higher-calorie food, or both. However we have little or no ways to understand how healthy is our food or what food items in the menu cater to our dietary requirements and restrictions. In addition to making a selection of healthy food, the cost of the selected menu item has to be within the budget. Therefore, consumers need help in selecting food item that fulfills following criteria: (i) right in calorie amount, (ii) contains ingredients that are beneficial for and absent of ingredients that are detrimental to individual health, and (iii) within a budget.

Our contribution in this research is three-fold. First, through a systematic literature review, we identify the research gap in smartphone-based dietary intervention technology. Second, we elicit the requirements of a system to address the research gaps. Third, we design and develop a dietary app for android platform that implements many of the elicited requirements.

2   Smartphone Application for Personal Health

Smartphones are equipped with embedded sensors such as acceleraometer, digital compass, gyroscope, GPS, microphone, camera, etc. Together with these sensors, smartphones provide a programmable platform for monitoring wellbeing as people go about their lives [3]. Smartphones also offer an effective software delivery channel such as popular Android marketplace or Apple app store.

Mobile devices can be used to make more informed decisions about health and wellness. According to Pew Internet and American Life Project survey [9], 19 per cent of smartphone users have at least one health app on their device. The survey also showed that 31 per cent of mobile phone owners have used their phones to look up health information.The survey also found that exercise, diet, and weight features are the most popular type of health apps downloaded. Ruder Finn[3] report found that among respondents of 1000 who say they use a health app, nearly half (49%) use healthy eating apps. Most of the existing mobile health apps focus on diet(e.g., [8]), physical activity (e.g., [1]), and stress (e.g., [7]).

Targeted towards weight loss, there are several popular diet-related apps, such as MyFitnessPal (myfitnesspal.com) and LiveStrong (livestrong. com) or Weight Watchers (weightwatchers.com). Balance [1] monitors the balance between caloric intake (user input based on the consumption of food) and caloric expenditure (based on daily activities). Calorie Tracker [10] is a diet and workout-tracking tool. The app tracks users diet, weight change, and workout to help people stay fit. The user enters the food consumed and the *LoseIt* app subtracts the caloric amount of the food from the total calories allowed per day. *LoseIt!*[4] app helps a user set a daily calorie budget, track food and exercise to achieve their weight goal.

---

[3] http://www.ruderfinn.com/
[4] http://www.loseit.com/what-is-lose-it/

The existing apps provide users with various types of feedback and information, such as exercise output, calorie intake, nutritional intake, etc. However, these apps do not directly contribute to our research problem of away-from-home food selection that matches aforementioned criteria.

3 Gaps in Existing Apps

To the best of our literature survey, there is no personal health dietary app that targets out of home food consumption. As such our research targets food consumption in restaurant. The consumption of more processed and convenience store foods of larger portion sizes, and the higher amounts of saturated fats and sugars in the diet result in caloric imbalance [5].

Personal lifestyles contribute to the global increase of many diet-related chronic diseases and conditions such as obesity, hypertension, etc. One of the major shifts in lifestyles is the increasing consumption of foods and drinks out of home such as restaurant [3]. Various researchers have expressed their concerns over out of home food consumptions with regard to larger portion sizes [4], higher energy densities [5], or healthy food choices [6]. Studies consistently show that eating out of home is particularly associated with higher total energy intake in adults, intake of fat, and lower intake of micronutrients, particularly vitamin C, Calcium and iron [3].

An access to affordable food is a major issue for many for living a healthy life. Research by Aggarwal et al. [12] shows that the social gradient in diet quality may be explained by diet cost. Miller et al. [13] evaluate the psychology of unemployed food shoppers during a recession and found that while individuals knew characteristics of healthy food, they were only buying sale items or coupons items. Therefore, selecting a healthy dietary option on a budget is a non-trivial task. We have not found an app that help users select a healthy eat-out menu item on a budget.

4 System Requirements

The goal of our research is to design a smartphone-based dietary app for selecting healthy food in an away-from-home setting (e.g., restaurant, fast food store, etc.) within budget. This app will automatically monitor healthy food intake habit of a consumer from the record of their selections.

4.1 Platform

The goal of personal health is to put individuals at the center of their health. As a result personal health apps need to be available at user's fingertips, which make smartphones and other handheld devices ideal platforms. Today's smartphone platforms include Google Android, Apple iOS, RIM BlackBerry, Nokia Symbian, and Windows.

4.2   Intended Target Users

There are some healthcare apps that target only consumers. However, consumers' participation alone cannot effectively achieve the goals of personal health. We view that one of the essential roles of technology is to facilitate interaction among different stakeholders. In a smartphone-based personal health application, these stakeholders include consumers, family and friends of the consumers, service providers, and care providers.

4.3   Functional Requirements

There are three basic functional requirements of a dietary application: monitoring, sharing, and intervention.

Food Intake Monitoring. Recording of dietary intake is essential for the assessment of healthy food intake habit. A study shows that a significant reduction ($p < .01$) in BMI is related with adherence to self-monitoring of food intake [17]. Self-monitoring raises the awareness of what people consume [18]. Arsand et al. [14] found that one of the key factors to success and sustainability of the recording of food consumption was the mobility of the recording device [15]. In other words, a diet app needs to offer anytime, anywhere, and effortless recording of food intake.

Requirement- and Restriction-Based On-budget Food Selection. Dietary intervention can be immediate (e.g., what to eat for next meal) and long-term (e.g., what adjustment is required in the consumption pattern). One of the challenges in achieving the result of dietary intervention is adherence. For example, Dansinger et al.'s study [16] reveals that adherence to any weight loss diet can work. Personalization is at the center of personal health. Dietary requirements and restrictions vary individual to individual. Identifying individual diet is a dietary intervention of a sort.

Sharing of Food Consumption Data. Sharing of monitored food intake information among related parties such as caregivers allows the respected parties to devise a proper wellness evaluation and dietary intervention to health conditions. There is evidence that peer support enhances successful lifestyle interventions for childhood obesity [14]. It can be used in administering proper family or peer support such as positive reinforcement and constructive feedback. Sharing of monitored data between consumer and caregiver may require sharing information across device platforms.

4.4   Non-functional Requiremnts

Even though many smartphone apps get downloaded, the true usage is lot less. Many of the downloaded apps are quickly abandoned due to unmet non-functional requirements.

Use Experience. A positive use experience is absolutely necessary for users to keep using the app. The app needs to be easy to use. Memorability is another desired feature so that the app remembers user input from the past use. In the context of our application, it should remember the food restrictions the consumers used in the past or budget amount the user spent for a particular meal. User interface is an important factor too.

Privacy Preferences and Security Concerns. Some apps, for instance, want to know a person's location using the phone's GPS sensor, which may be perceived by users as a threat to their location privacy. Thirty percent of app users say they have removed an app once they found out how much information it collected about them [11]. While sharing information with other apps or across platform, a fine-grained access control policy needs to be enforced.

Food Service Providers' Policies. An away-from-home dietary application requires involvement of restaurants or food stores. This consumer-side app would include menu items from different restaurants and eateries. As a result, the app may also need to enforce policies of food service providers.

5 Implementation

Kalico consists of a client-side application connected to a remote database. The client-side app, written in Java, runs on Android devices. The initial version of the remote database executes on a MySQL server. All of the restaurant meal data is stored in a remote database which is accessed by this application.

There is a budgeting functionality with the program as well where the user can maintain a balance. This balance is stored on the mobile device in the SQLite database. When the user purchases a meal, its price is automatically deducted from their balance and information about the meal is stored in a log on their device. Kalico was written using the Java Android Development Tools (ADT) plugin for the Eclipse application development framework. The application requires Android 2.2 and above.

5.1 Design Diagram

The client-side application is composed of GUI and non-GUI elements. Each screen, known as an Activity, requires a separate class. Non-graphical functionality can occur in these classes or in other classes. The server-side application must return menu information in an XML format. Kalico consists of the following components:

1. Update Criteria (executes on smartphone): Present user with GUI for gathering meal criteria.
2. Make Request (executes on smartphone): Translate user criteria into format suitable for building a query to the remote database.
3. Query to Server (executes on smartphone): After building the query, it will send query from server to the database.
4. PHP Retrieve Data (executes on server): Retrieve query results from the database and translate XML format.
5. Data Parser (executes on smartphone): Translates XML data into a meal object. Iterates over all data until all objects are created.
6. Update Balance of User (executes on smartphone): SQLite component that will update balance of the user on the local device.
7. Log of Meals (executes on smartphone): Update the tables in the local database from meal object selected.

Figure 1 illustrates the interaction between the various components. The graphical user interaction is through the Update Criteria, Log of Meals, and Update User Balance components.

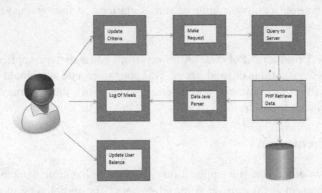

Fig. 1. Kalico Component Architecture

5.2   Screenshots

Kalico is composed of 10 screens.

Launch Screen serves as the entry point for the application. User can see their current balance, add/subtract from their balance, view history and health tips, or search for meals.

Update Balance Screen allows the user to add or subtract money from their balance. A balance must be entered in order to utilize the balance feature.

Restaurant Selection Activity allows the user to select a restaurant. Restaurants are grouped alphabetically in a collapsible list. Selecting a restaurant takes the user to the Criteria Selection Screen.

Criteria Selection Screen allows the user to specify the elements of the criteria of their meals. Selected elements will be included in the user search. Pressing *Submit* takes the user to Criteria Restriction Screen.

Criteria Restriction Screen allows the user to specify the restrictions on the selected criteria. Only the items selected on Criteria Selection Screen will be available for restriction. Pressing *Submit* takes the user to the Meal Parts Selection Screen. The user must enter a restriction for all selected criteria.

Meal Parts Selection Screen allows the user to specify the parts of a meal to include (e.g. entre, side item, beverage, etc). Pressing Submit initiates the request for meals to be returned from the server.

Meal Query Results Screen shows summaries of the meal results of the query in a list. Selecting a meal takes the user to the Meal Confirmation Screen.

Meal Confirmation Screen presents the user with details of the selected meal. Here, the user sees the items of the meal, price, and all nutritional information. The user can confirm this selection, or can return to the Meal Query Results Screen by selecting the Back button. If the user does confirm the selection, the price of the meal is subtracted from the balance and the user is returned to the Launch Screen.

View History Screen presents the user with the history of all selected meals. Pressing the Clear History button erases the meal history and returns the user to the Launch Screen.

Health Tips Activity presents the user with nutritional health tips. The information is categorized based on Calories, Sugar, Fat, Sodium, Protein, and Carbs. The information is presented in an expandable list.

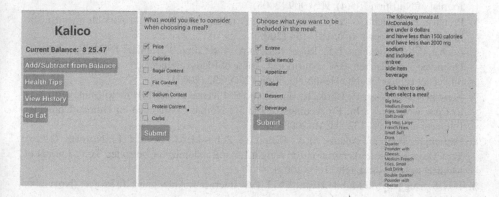

Fig. 2. Kalico Screenshots

6   Discussions

The current shifts in modern lifestyles causes many people to eat outside of the home. The menu choices available are typically less healthy, and more costly, than food made in the home. The consumption of less healthy foods leads to chronic ailments such as diabetes and hypertension.

We have presented Kalico as a tool that allows users to quickly identify healthy meals at restaurants that satisfy nutritional and budgetary requirements. Kalico also explains the benefits and drawbacks of eating different food items .

An initial implementation of Kalico has been uploaded into the marketplace. Kalico app has been in Android marketplace for about two weeks. Currently, there are over 60 downloads. It has received 13 reviews with an average of 3.9 out of 5 stars. User feedback validates the usefulness of the app, as well as suggests methods for improvement. This feedback will be incorporated into future releases of Kalico.

References

1. Denning, T., Andrew, A., Chaudhri, R., Hartung, C., Lester, J., Borriello, G., Duncan, G.: Balance: Towards a Usable Pervasive Wellness Application with Accurate Activity Inference. In: Proceedings of the 10th Workshop on Mobile Computing Systems and Applications, p. 5. ACM (2009)
2. Lane, N.D., Mohammod, M., Lin, M., Yang, X., Lu, H., Ali, S., Campbell, A.: Bewell: A smartphone application to monitor, model and promote wellbeing. In: 5th International Conference on Pervasive Computing Technologies for Healthcare (2011)
3. Lachat, C., Nago, E., Verstraeten, R., Roberfroid, D., Van Camp, J., Kolsteren, P.: Eating out of home and its association with dietary intake: a systematic review of the evidence. Obesity Reviews 13(4), 329–346 (2012)
4. Ledikwe, J.H., Ello-Martin, J.A., Rolls, B.J.: Portion sizes and the obesity epidemic. The Journal of Nutrition 135(4), 905–909 (2005)
5. Prentice, A.M., Jebb, S.A.: Fast foods, energy density and obesity: a possible mechanistic link. Obesity Reviews 4(4), 187–194 (2003)
6. Lachat, C.K., Huybregts, L.F., Roberfroid, D.A., Van Camp, J., Remaut-De Winter, A.M.E., Debruyne, P., Kolsteren, P.W.: Nutritional profile of foods offered and consumed in a Belgian university canteen. Public Health Nutrition 12(1), 122 (2009)
7. Ferreira, P., Sanches, P., Höök, K., Jaensson, T.: License to chill!: How to Empower Users to Cope with Stress. In: Proceedings of the 5th Nordic Conference on Human-Computer Interaction, pp. 123–132. ACM (2008)
8. Patrick, K., Raab, F., Adams, M.A., Dillon, L., Zabinski, M., Rock, C.L., Norman, G.J.: A Text Message based Intervention for Weight Loss: Randomized Controlled Trial. Journal of Medical Internet Research 11(1) (2009)
9. Fox, S., Duggan, M.: Mobile Health 2012. Pew Internet & American Life Project (November 8, 2012)
10. Kim, H., Kim, T., Joo, M., Yi, S., Yoo, C., Lee, K., Chung, G.: Design of a Calorie Tracker Utilizing Heart Rate Variability Obtained by a Nanofiber Technique-based Wellness Wear System. Applied Mathematics and Information Science, Special Issue 5(2), 70–73 (2011)
11. Boyles, J.L., Smith, A., Madden, M.: Privacy and Data Management on Mobile Devices. Pew Internet & American Life Project (Sepetenber 5, 2012),
http://pewinternet.org/Reports/2012/Mobile-Privacy/Main-Findings/Section-1.aspx
12. Aggarwal, A., Monsivais, P., Cook, A.J., Drewnowski, A.: Does Diet Cost Mediate the Relation between Socio-economic Position and Diet Quality & Quest. European Journal of Clinical Nutrition 65(9), 1059–1066 (2011)
13. Miller, C.K., Branscum, P.: The Effect of a Recessionary Economy on Food Choice: Implications for Nutrition Education. Journal of Nutrition Education and Behavior 44(2), 100–106 (2012)
14. Arsand, E., Tufano, J.T., Ralston, J.D., Hjortdahl, P.: Designing Mobile Dietary Management Support Technologies for People with Diabetes. Journal of Telemedicine and Telecare 14(7), 329–332 (2008)
15. Phillips, G., Felix, L., Galli, L., Patel, V., Edwards, P.: The effectiveness of M-health Technologies for Improving Health and Health Services: A Systematic Review Protocol. BMC Research Notes 3(1), 250 (2010)
16. Dansinger, M.L., Gleason, J.A., Griffith, J.L., Selker, H.P., Schaefer, E.J.: Comparison of the Atkins, Ornish, Weight Watchers, and Zone Diets for Weight Loss and Heart Disease Risk Reduction. JAMA: the Journal of the American Medical Association 293(1), 43–53 (2005)

17. Jelalian, E., Lloyd-Richardson, E.E., Mehlenbeck, R.S., Hart, C.N., Flynn-O'Brien, K., Kaplan, J., Neill, M., Wing, R.R.: Behavioral Weight Control Treatment with Supervised Exercise or Peer-enhanced Adventure for Overweight Adolescents. The Journal of Pediatrics 157(6), 923–928 (2010)
18. Wadden, T.A., Foster, G.D.: Behavioral treatment of obesity. Medical Clinics of North America 84(2), 441–461 (2000)
19. Guthrie, J.F., Lin, B.H., Frazao, E.: Role of Food Prepared Away from Home in the American Diet, 1977-78 versus 1994-96: Changes and Consequences. Journal of Nutrition Education and Behavior 34(3), 140–150 (2002)

Walk Route Recommendation for Fitness Walkers Using Calorie Consumption Prediction

Yuki Sakon, Hung-Hsuan Huang, and Kyoji Kawagoe

Ritsumeikan University,
Kusatsu-city, Shiga, Japan
sakon@coms.ritsumei.ac.jp, huang@fc.ritsumei.ac.jp,
kawagoe@is.ritsumei.ac.jp

Abstract. In this paper, we propose a novel method for recommendation of a walking route for fitness walkers, effective for health maintenance. Recently, lifestyle-related disease has been increasing in the world. It is important for people to keep balance between the calorie intake and the calorie consumption. We focus on calorie consumption by walking. Walking is effective exercise for maintaining and promoting healthy life. It is necessary to select a walking route where calorie consumption makes effectively. We propose a method of the recommendation of the walking route which can use an effective calorie in consideration of the characteristic of the user. The method is mainly composed of two features: prediction of calorie consumption and search of an appropriate walking route. Some evaluation results of our method are also described in the paper.

Keywords: METS, Time series, Health science, Calorie prediction, Walking Support.

1 Introduction

The world has recently witnessed an increase in the incidence of lifestyle-related diseases such as hypertension, hyperlipidemia, and diabetes. It is important for people to maintain a balance between their calorie intake and calories consumed. Walking is effective exercise for maintaining and promoting healthy life. The U. S. Centers for Disease Control and Prevention recommends at least 150 minutes of moderate-intensity walking exercise each week [1]. This amount of exercise equals 30 minutes of exercise five days each week. However, even if we walk at the same time, calorie consumption values vary with route elevation and walkers walking characteristics. If we could select a walking route in order to consume calorie effectively, we can better improve access to health care. There is a web service that can easily calculate calorie consumption with the input of the total distance walked [2]. However, the accuracy of this method implemented in this web service, is poor because it does not take into account the walker's gait, which varies considerably between individuals, and the path elevation. In order to select a walking route for effective calorie consumption, we realize an accurate prediction of calorie consumption before walking.

D. Zeng et al. (Eds.): ICSH 2013, LNCS 8040, pp. 122–133, 2013.

In this paper, we propose a novel method of predicting calorie consumption for "fitness walkers" before walking and also propose a method of recommending a new route enabling the maximum calorie consumption per unit-time. The spot of the proposed method is to search the previous routes similar to the data from the current route according to the similarity in the path gradient and the walker's gait, used for calorie consumption prediction. With use of this route searching, more accurate prediction can be realized. Moreover, the point of the new route recommendation is to find the route between the current spot and the destination with the maximum calorie consumption per unit time.

2   Related Work

Several important research studies [3][4][5][6], with the help of computer technology, have been performed on the prevention of lifestyle-related disease. Kozakai et al. proposed a wearable dietary and health information logging system, composed of a cellular phone, a sphygmomanometer, a body composition monitor, and a calorie consumption meter [7]. They have also conducted an experiment with a male subject and obtained his dietary and health information continuously for a month. Sumida et al. suggested a health-conscious walking navigation system that recommends a walking route with minimal perceived exertion satisfying the constraints of calorie consumption and walking time [8]. For effective and continuous walking, a walking route must be selected manually that is suitable for an individual's physical ability. Though perceived exertion during walking can be estimated by monitoring the heart rate, it is costly for an individual to use a special device such as a heart rate monitor. They built a perceived exertion model that predicts the heart rate from walking data, including acceleration and walking speed, in order to estimate perceived exertion during walking with the available smartphone functions. Although these studies have been done so far, there still exists a crucial issue on effective exercise to be solved.

3   Walking Route Recommendation

In this section, we describe some definitions on the walking route and the methods of calorie consumption prediction as well as of walking route recommendation.

3.1   Defintions

A walking route is defined as a path between a start spot and the goal spot. The walking route includes attitude and distance information. The walking route is represented by a trajectory which is a temporal sequence of <distance, elevation>.

A Metabolic Equivalent Task (MET) is a measure of exercise intensity [10]. METs are directly related to the intensity of physical activity and the amount of oxygen consumed. The larger the MET value the more is the amount of calories burned. Exercise physiologists use METs to determine what activity is appropriate for people according to their current fitness level. One MET is equal to the amount of oxygen consumed at rest, and 2 METs means that twice the amount of oxygen is needed for a particular activity than is needed at rest. Ainsworth et al. defined the METs for each exercise [9]. The amount of calories burned can easily be calculated using the MET values and the equation proposed by the American College of Sports Medicine (ACSM) [10]. The calorie consumption value is a function of the MET/h value and the subject's body weight, as shown in the equation below.

$$Calorie\ Consumption(kcal) = 1.05 \cdot Mets \cdot hours \cdot body\ weight(kg) \qquad (1)$$

Lastly, we explain here the User Action State Database, called UAS database. The following three information is stored in UAS database:

- H: Elevation (m): Elevation time series data is acquired from GPS.
- K: Distance (m): Distance data is acquired and calculated from the degree of latitude and longitude by using Hubeny's distance formula [12].
- Activity intensity (METs): Exercise intensity data is acquired from 3-axis accelerometer data.

3.2   Issues to Be Solved

As mentioned previously, calorie consumption values vary with route elevation and subject's walking characteristics. Although it is important to account for these factors, it is also difficult to do so because of the following two main factors.

- Elevation
  More calories are burned while jogging uphill than jogging on a flat road, because the former involves a greater effort. An FAA study reported the results of the measurement of calories burned while jogging at 9 mph on 3 surfaces. A 205 pound person burned 1,269 calories per hour, or 141 calories per mile, on a level surface [11]. However, the same person burned 1,480 calories per hour, or 164 calories per mile, on a 2.5% uphill gradient. While jogging on a 4% uphill gradient, the subject burned 1,564 calories in an hour, or 174 calories per mile. A 125-pound person burned 86, 101, and 107 calories per mile on a level surface, on a small gradient, and on a larger gradient, respectively. We also tested to show the relationship between calorie consumption and walking speed in a male subject walking at constant speed on different gradients. Table 1 shows our findings, which shows that calorie consumption varies according to route elevation.
- Walking characteristics
  Calorie consumption varies from individual to individual. We measured the difference in calorie consumption in two subjects. Two young males walked

Table 1. Calorie consumption while walking at different speeds

Slope	0 percent slope	7.5 percent slope	15 percent slope
	420 kcal	448 kcal	560 kcal

simultaneously on the same path and at the same constant speed. We calculated the calories burned using a calorie calculator and a 3-axes accelerometer. Fig. 1 shows the results. Please note that METs are used instead of calories because the equipment can measure METs for calorie calculation. The findings showed that the METs of subjects 1 and 2 were different, although temporal trends of METs of both may have been similar. Calorie consumption of subject 1 was greater than that of subject 2.

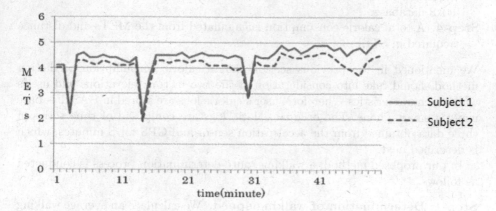

Fig. 1. Walking characteristic

Therefore, the basic ideas of our proposed prediction method to solve the above issues are described here.

The method is mainly composed of two features: calorie consumption prediction and selection of the route. We extract and store calorie logs of walking activities in a format of time series, beforehand. Before walking exercise, time series of the past routes which are all similar to the time series of the walking route are searched with use of peculiarity similarity definition. The calorie consumption is estimated from these past walking time series.

Moreover, a start spot and the goal spot are decided in the determination of walking route beforehand. There are candidate walking routes in the goal spot from a start spot. We predict calories consumption and the walking speed of the candidate walking route. We recommend for the most efficient walking route severely in a candidate route.

3.3   Prediction and Route Recommendation

We provide the predicted calorie consumption to the user as described in the following steps. Then, we explain the process of route recommendation.

We collect walking data with the smartphone. Then, we store these time series in the UAS database. We compute a user's METs by using a 3-axis accelerometer and acquire the position time series data for the user's walk from the user's past movement. We extract the METs in the position time series data in every $\triangle T$ minutes.

Step-1. The predicted walking speed is obtained from UAS database.

Step-2. Elevation time series data and predicted distance after every S min are calculated with regard to the predicted walking speed.

Step-3. The similarity with the User Action State (UAS) database's elevation time series data is calculated. Then, using the K-nearest neighbor (K-NN) algorithm the average METs and the average distance are obtained from the UAS database.

Step-4. A total calorie consumption is calculated from the METs and distance acquired in STEP-3.

We mentioned in the previous section that a calorie consumption prediction method should take into consideration of the two factors: elevations and user's walking characteristics. Therefore, user's calorie logs are stored in UAS database using a smart phone. The original calorie logs are composed of time series of three data obtained from the acceleration sensor and GPS for S minutes, which is described next.

In our proposed method, a walking route determination process is conducted as follows:

Step-1: Determination of walking speed. We calculate an average walking speed from UAS database.

Step-2: Search of the candidate route. We search the candidate routes more than N to a start spot and the goal spot .

Step-3: Calorie consumption prediction. We calculate predictive calorie consumption using the above Step-3 method.

Step-4 : Determination of recommendation walking route. We calculate a weight between two spots , called *E-value*, using predicted calorie consumption and predicted walking time.

As a start spot and the goal spot are decided in the determination of walking route, we select the most suitable walking route from some walking routes. We define the efficiency degree as *E-value* by an efficient walking route. The *E-value* of the route between two spots is a function of the predicted calorie consumption and predicted walking time, as shown in the equation below.

$$E - value = (predicted\ calorie\ consumption)/(predicted\ walking\ time) \quad (2)$$

We select the walking route which can carry out calorie consumption of the user more efficiently from the candidate walking routes for two spots.

3.4   Example

The calorie consumption while walking from A spot to B spot is not the same
as that when walking from B to A, if there is a gradient between points A and
B. This difference is because more energy is needed for walking uphill than for
walking downhill, even if the same route is taken between points A and B. Another difficulty in predicting calorie consumption stems from user characteristics,
usually an expenditure of energy while walking differs from person to person,
even if the individuals walk on the same road at the same speed. We set A as
a start point and set B to the end spots. We extract four candidate walking
routes between A and B and represent the four routes by Route 1, Route 2,
Route 3, Route 4. We calculate an average walking speed from UAS database.
Elevation time series data and predicted distances after every S minutes are calculated with regard to the predicted walking speed. We assume a walking speed
to be 6km per hour, S=5 and K=2. Then, The similarity with elevation time
series data in the UAS database is calculated every 500m. Then, the 2-nearest
neighbor algorithm (2-NN) the average METs and distance are obtained from
the UAS database. We calculate predictive calorie consumption using suggestion
technique in the walking route. We calculate *E-value* between two spots using
predicted calorie consumption and predicted walking time.

Table 2 shows our findings. It shows the distance, the predictive calorie consumption, the predictive walk time and *E-value* for each route. Then, we can
recommend a Route 3 whose *E-value* is the largest among the four routes.

Table 2. Example

	Route 1	Route 2	Route 3	Route 4
Distance	6600m	7300m	7100m	5000m
Predicted calorie consumption	435kcal	580 kcal	560 kcal	344kcal
Predicted walking time	49mim	66min	50min	33min
E-value	8.8	8.7	11.2	10.4

3.5   Proposed Methods of Predicting Calorie and of Route Recommendation

Finding Similar Past Walking Routes

The biggest challenge here is to predict calorie consumption for a new, unknown,
walking route. As described previously, the two factors, the route elevation and
the user characteristics have a strong effect on calorie consumption. Although
the start and the end spots of a particular day's walking are fixed, there may be
many possible routes between the two spots. Moreover, owing to varying path
elevations along a route, the estimated calorie consumption may vary considerably from the actual calorie consumption.

In order to predict calorie consumption for a new path that takes the two factors into account, we first obtain the amount of calories to be consumed for the next P minutes from the current time. All the calorie consumption values that had been predicted up to current time for each $P \times S$ minute interval were collected and added. The route for $P \times S$ minutes is called a route segment. Each route consists of small route segments. It is assumed the time interval of a route segment is constant, S minutes. Route l_j is a sequence of route segments, $route \; l_j = < e1, e2, e3, ... >$. We obtain the previous route that is most similar to the new route by using the following distance definitions d(l_{new},l_{log}), the distance between a new route l_{new} and one of the past routes l_{log} as follows.

$$d(l_{new}, l_{log}) = \Sigma_j |\triangle Elevation(e_{new,j}) - \triangle Elevation(e_{log,j})| \tag{3}$$

where $e_{new,j}$ and $e_{log,j}$ are route segments for a log route and a new route, respectively. $\triangle Elevation(e_k)$ is the difference between the elevation of the start spot and the elevation of the end spot for route segment e_k.

Calorie Consumption Prediction Using K-NN

According to the above definition of distance, the K most similar routes can be found by a K-NN search. After getting the routes by a K-NN search from the UAS database, the average calorie consumption values for the different routes are calculated and the predicted calorie consumption values are tabulated. The total predicted calorie consumption is calculated by adding all the predicted calorie consumption numbers for the route segments. The calorie consumption for a route is calculated using the equation proposed by the American College of Sports Medicine [10]. It can also be determined using an hourly MET value and the user's weight.

Waking Route Recommendation

We propose a method of the recommendation of the walking route using an effective calorie in consideration of the characteristic of the user. In Figure 2, our method architecture is depicted. First, we search the candidate route to a start spot and the goal spot more than N. Then, we calculate predictive calorie consumption using suggestion technique in the walking route. We extract a candidate walking route from Google Maps. The candidate walking route is assumed to be a route using a pedestrian precinct and the sidewalk on foot a candidate route in Google Maps and acquires elevation data. Afterword, we calculate the E value using predicted calorie consumption and predicted walking time. Finally, We can recommend the top K from a route the candidate route.

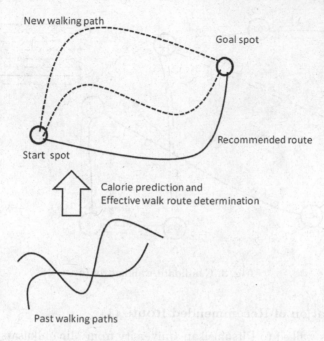

Fig. 2. Our method architecture

4 Evaluations

4.1 Setup

Five subjects stored their UAS database in their smartphones for 7 days and acquired the elevation time series data of total 360 minutes during 7 days. We consider a crossing of the route as node. We connected the shortest distance between nodes and found all the routes as candidate routes.

4.2 Experiments

We set Minami-kusatsu station as the start spot and set Ritsumeikan University to the end spot. We performed two experiments: the experiment on recommended routes and the experiment on accuracy of calorie consumption prediction. The results of these two experiments are described below.

In these experiments, we compared our results with the existing system called Kyorisoku web services. Kyorisoku is a web service that can easily calculate calorie consumption with the input of the total distance walked. It does not take into account the walker's gait, which varies considerably between individuals and the path elevation.

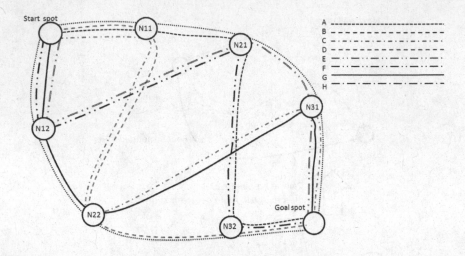

Fig. 3. Candidate walking route

4.3   Evaluation of Recommended Route (1)

Five subjects walked to Ritsumeikan University from Minamikusatsu at an approximately constant speed (6 km/h), the walking distance one-way was about 3,300 m and the difference in elevation was 52 m. We predicted the calorie consumption for a new unknown walking route by using both our method and the kyorisoku web service [2].

We calculate *E-value* between two spots using predicted calorie consumption and predicted walking time. We also calculate the each modulus as correct answer data of real *E-values*.

We used the following recommended route's appropriateness (RRA) formula for evaluation. This number indicates that the smaller one has good appropriation.

$$RRA = \frac{1}{N} \times \Sigma_i \frac{|Predicted_{E-value(i)} - Actual_{E-value(i)}|}{Actual_{E-value(i)}} \tag{4}$$

where $Predicted_{E-value(i)}$ is a predicted value of *E-value* for $subject_i$. $Actual_{E-value(i)}$ is an actual value of *E-value* for $subject_i$, and N is the number of subjects.

Table 3 and 4 show the results of this evaluation. As shown in Table 4, the RRA was about 0.051 for our method and about 0.293 for the kyorisoku system.

Therefore, the recommended route's appropriateness of our method is better than the existing web service.

4.4   Evaluation of Recommended Route (2)

We extract the following routes from these a candidate walking route. Fig. 3 shows the candidate walking routes.

Table 3. Results of the *E-value*

	Actual *E-value*	Our method	Kyorisoku
Subject 1	9.61	10.1	7.50
Subject 2	7.48	7.45	5.35
Subject 3	6.31	5.92	4.43
Subject 4	6.63	6.29	4.96
Subject 5	7.2	6.57	4.21

Table 4. Results of RRA

	Our method	Kyorisoku
RRA	0.051	0.293

Route A=< $N11, N21, N31$ >, Route B=< $N11, N21, N32$ >, Route C=< $N11, N22, N31$ >, Route D=< $N11, N22, N32$ >, Route E=< $N12, N21, N31$ >, Route F=< $N12, N21, N32$ >, Route G=< $N12, N22, N31$ >, and Route H=< $N12, N22, N32$ >. N_k is a node representing a crossing with in the subject's walking route.

Then we calculate the calorie consumption prediction and walking time of these ways. We recommended the route of three high ranks. Table 5 shows the our method and kyorisoku results of this experiment. From the Table 5, it is obvious that the recommended routes were different individually by our method. On the other hand, All the recommended routes by the kyorisoku system are the same.

Therefore, our method can recommend the walking route which can use an effective calorie in consideration of the characteristic of the user, more accurate than the existing system.

Table 5. Top 3 routes

	Our method	Kyorisoku
Subject1	A,F,E	D,E,G
Subject2	A,E,D	D,E,G
Subject3	A,B,D	D,E,G
Subject4	A,B,E	D,E,G
Subject5	B,A,E	D,E,G

4.5 Accuracy of Calorie Consumption Prediction

Five subjects walked from Ritsumeikan University to Minamikusatsu station (Biwako-Kusatsu Campus, Japan) at an approximately constant speed once a day. The walking distance was about 3,300 m and the difference in elevation was 48 m. We used the following prediction accuracy (PA) formula for evaluation.

$$PA = (1 - |Predicted\ calorie - Consumed\ calorie|/Consumed\ calorie) \times 100(\%)$$
$$(5)$$

Calorie consumption prediction was performed every minute after the user began the walk. Table 6 shows the results from this experiment. It shows from the Table 6 that the average of accuracy obtained using our method was 94.1% and 91.9%. The average of kyorisoku was 86.7% and 82.0%.

Therefore, it is confirmed that our method was better than the existing method. This accuracy appears to be sufficient to provide a credible numerical values of calorie consumption.

Table 6. Results of evaluation of prediction accuracy (PA)

Average		PA (Sta. to Univ.)		PA (Univ. to Sta.)	
		Our method	Kyorisoku	Our method	PA Kyorisoku
Subject 1	55kg	89.7	80.0	87.3	76.9
Subject 2	65kg	94.2	93.5	89.5	86.9
Subject 3	58kg	92.5	93.0	94.7	88.8
Subject 4	82kg	94.4	86.0	95.9	80.8
Subject 5	70kg	99.9	81.2	92.0	76.9
Average		94.1	86.7	91.9	82.0

5 Conclusions

In this paper, we propose a novel method for recommendation of a walking route for fitness walkers, effective for health maintenance. Our method can recommend the walking route which can use an effective calorie in consideration of the characteristic of the user. The accuracy seems to be enough to obtain credible numerical values for calorie consumption.

We need to improve the accuracy in prediction calorie consumption and recommend walking route. In the future, we plan to perform more detailed and subjective evaluations. Further, we will develop a prototype system for real-time walking route recommendation for nutritional energy control on the basis of the nutritional energy awareness concepts.

Acknowledgement. This work was partially supported by JSPS KAKENHI Grant Number 24300039. We would like to thank Professor Kiyoshi Sanada and Professor Motoyuki Iemitsu for giving us a great deal of information on sports and health science.

References

1. Centers for Disease Control and Prevention, http://www.cdc.gov/
2. Kyorisoku Powered By Mapion, http://www.mapion.co.jp/route/
3. Lara, O.D., Perez, A.J., Labrador, M.A., Posada, J.D.: Centinela: A human activity recognition system based on acceleration and vital sign data. Journal on Pervasive and Mobile Computing (2011)
4. Varshney, U.: Pervasive Healthcare and Wireless Health Monitoring. ACM/Baltzer Journal of Mobile Networks and Applications 12(2-3), 113–127 (2007)
5. Zhao, N.: Full-Featured Pedometer. Design Realized with 3-Axis. Digital Accelerometer Analog Dialogue 44(6), 1–5 (2010)
6. Kawahara, Y., Ryu, N., Asami, T.: Monitoring Daily Energy Expenditure using a 3-Axis Accelerometer with a Low-Power Microprocessor. International Journal on Human-Computer Interaction 1(5), 145–154 (2009)
7. Kozakai, K., Tanigichi, S., Fukuda, T., Nakauchi, Y.: Dietary and Health Information Logging System for Lifestyle-Related Diseases. In: IEEE Conf. on Information Acquisition, pp. 829–834 (2006)
8. Sumida, M., Imazu, S., Mizumot, T., Yasumoto, K.: Estimation of Perceived Exertion using Smartphone for Health-Conscious Walking Navigation. IPSJ SIG Technical Report, Vol.2012-MBL-62, 1-8 (2012) (in Japanese)
9. Ainsworth, B.E., Haskell, W.L., Whitt, M.C., Irwin, M.L., Swartz, A.M., Strath, S.J., O'Brien, W.L., Bassett Jr., D.R., Schmitz, K.H., Emplaincourt, P.O., Jacobs Jr., D.R., Leon, A.S.: Compendium of Physical Activities: an update of activity codes and MET intensities. Med. Sci. Sports Exerc. 32, S498–S504 (2000)
10. American College of Sports Medicine, http://www.acsm.org/
11. Federal Aviation Administration, http://www.faa.gov/
12. Haraki, T., Yokoyama, S., Fukuta, N., Ishikawa, H.: On Generating Tag about Moving Object Using GPS Location Data and Web Resources. DEIM Forum, B8–B5 (2011) (in Japanese)

AZDrugMiner: An Information Extraction System for Mining Patient-Reported Adverse Drug Events in Online Patient Forums

Xiao Liu and Hsinchun Chen

MIS Department, University of Arizona, Tucson, United States
xiaoliu@email.arizona.edu, hchen@eller.arizona.edu

Abstract. Post-marketing drug surveillance is a critical component of drug safety. Drug regulatory agencies such as the U.S. Food and Drug Administration (FDA) rely on voluntary reports from health professionals and consumers contributed to its FDA Adverse Event Reporting System (FAERS) to identify adverse drug events (ADEs). However, it is widely known that FAERS underestimates the prevalence of certain adverse events. Popular patient social media sites such as DailyStrength and PatientsLikeMe provide new information sources from which patient-reported ADEs may be extracted. In this study, we propose an analytical framework for extracting patient-reported adverse drug events from online patient forums. We develop a novel approach – the AZDrugMiner system – based on statistical learning to extract ad-verse drug events in patient discussions and identify reports from patient experiences. We evaluate our system using a set of manually annotated forum posts which show promising performance. We also examine correlations and differences between patient ADE reports extracted by our system and reports from FAERS. We conclude that patient social media ADE reports can be extracted effectively using our proposed framework. Those patient reports can reflect unique perspectives in treatment and be used to improve patient care and drug safety.

Keywords: Patient Forums, Adverse Drug Events, Information Extraction, Health Social Media Analytics, Health Big Data.

1 Introduction

It is estimated that approximately 2 million patients in the United States are affected each year by adverse drug events (ADEs), making adverse drug event the fourth leading cause of death in the U.S. [5]. The responsibility of post-marketing drug safety within the United States lies with the Food and Drug Administration (FDA), part of the U.S. Department of Health and Human Services. The information related to adverse drug events (ADEs) is reported to the FDA's Adverse Event Reporting System (FAERS) [9] by healthcare professionals, pharmaceutical companies and health consumers. However, it is widely known that FAERS underestimates the prevalence of certain adverse events [5].

D. Zeng et al. (Eds.): ICSH 2013, LNCS 8040, pp. 134–150, 2013.
© Springer-Verlag Berlin Heidelberg 2013

Social media sites have become ubiquitous, and many new patient-centric online discussion forums and social websites, such as PatientsLikeMe [21] and Daily-Strength [9], have emerged as platforms for supporting patient discussions of diseases and treatments. These patient social platforms also attract the attention of researchers and health professionals. Of particular interest are patients' accounts of their experiences with drug treatments. Patient accounts come from a large and diverse population and may provide valuable supplementary information for drug safety regulatory agencies [2]. The adverse events discussed in social media can also reflect underlying reasons for patient's drug non-compliance [14]. However, extracting patient-reported adverse drug events still faces several challenges. Topics in patient social media come from various sources, including news and research, stories of patients' experiences, and third-hand accounts. Redundant and noisy information often masks patient-experienced ADEs. Also, current approaches extracting adverse event and drug relation in patient comments result in low precision and accuracy, particularly in sentences with multiple drugs and events [2]. A more robust approach to identifying adverse drug events would be of great asset to improving healthcare.

In this paper, we develop and evaluate an analytical framework (AZDrugMiner) for extracting patient-reported adverse drug events from online patient forums. We propose to identify drug-event associations more precisely through the application of machine learning-based relation extraction and by extracting ADE reports based on true patient experiences. Moreover, we anticipate that patient social media ADE reports show different perspectives in drug safety surveillance provide health professionals with a better understanding of patients' needs, facilitate personalized healthcare and improve patient safety.

The remainder of the paper is organized as follows. Section 2 provides a review of relevant literature and identifies potential research gaps. Section 3 presents our proposed AZDrugMiner framework. Section 4 describes our dataset and experiment setting, and discusses the results. Finally, section 5 concludes the study and identifies future directions.

2   Related Work

To form the basis of our research, we review the prior studies that emphasize mining user comments in patient social media. We develop a review of previous studies based on data source, research focus, text mining techniques, and performance.

2.1   Data Sources in Patient Social Media Research

A large number of patient social media platforms are available on the Internet and present different characteristics. Prior studies have explored general health discussion forums, such as DailyStrength [13][18], MedHelp [26] and health forums in Yahoo! Groups [4]; disease-focused discussion forums such as breastcancer.org, komen.org, and csn.cancer.org [2]; and micro blogs (Twitter) [3]. General health discussion forums contain a wide range of topics from herbal remedies to medication experiences. User comments from those forums require noise filtering before further analysis [5]. Disease-focused discussion forums contain more concentrated treatment discussions and disease-relevant patient profiles, presenting great potential for generating medical hypotheses [2]. Twitter uses short sentences ("tweets" of 140 or fewer characters); patients sometimes indicate their drug use and associated side effects on Twitter and present real-time information useful for pharmacovigilance [3]. Overall, mining these disease-focused discussion forums for adverse drug event reports is promising as they contain less noise, more concentrated treatment discussions, and better documented patient profile information.

2.2   Health Focus of Prior Patient Social Media Research

Many different analyses can be performed with patient social media data such as extracting adverse drug events, drug outcome analysis, etc. A major focus of prior patient social media research has been to extract adverse events from patient forums [2][3][13][18][26]. Other focuses of prior studies have included mining patient opinion toward treatments to identify risky drugs on the market [5] and extracting drug outcomes from patient forums to help patients better understand their treatments [10].

2.3   Text Mining Techniques

The most commonly adopted text mining techniques in patient social media research include text classification, medical entity recognition, and entity relation extraction. In this section, we discuss these techniques and their applications in the healthcare context.

Text Classification

A common problem in patient social media is noisy data. Filtering noise and extracting relevant data for analysis are important processes [2]. Text classification has been applied in patient social forums to filter noise [3] and to classify positive or negative drug effects [5]. Support Vector Machines (SVM), one of the most popular text classification techniques, has been widely adopted in patient social media research [2, 3]. Although many text classifiers have been developed in past studies, none of them has focused on distinguishing news or hearsay (i.e., other people's stories) from patients' own experiences.

Named Entity Recognition and Extraction

In the context of patient social media, researchers need to extract user comments related to drugs and adverse events. Named entity recognition is a common way to accomplish this. The process of named entity recognition refers to the task of finding spans of text that constitute proper names and then classifying the entities according to their type. In the healthcare-related context, it enables recognition of terms denoting specific classes (e. g., drugs and adverse events) in patient discussions.

Most studies adopt lexicon-based entity extraction approaches because of the wide availability of medical lexicons in the healthcare domain. Many different knowledge bases and dictionaries have been applied to the construction of lexicons in prior studies. Standard medical knowledge bases such as Unified Medical Language System (UMLS) [25] have been adopted in prior studies to extract drug name entities [2][5][13]. Drug safety databases have also been used to extract adverse event entities from patient forums [3][5][13]. Those databases include: MedEffect [16], a drug safety surveillance database in Canada; FAERS, the adverse event reporting system for the U.S.; and SIDER [11], a database used for medication package inserts. Recent studies have also adopted the Consumer Health Vocabulary (CHV) [5], a lexicon linking UMLS standard medical terms to health consumer vocabulary, to better understand and match users' expressions in social media [2][25].

Other studies have adopted a machine learning approach. Nikfarjam et al. [18] used association rule mining to find patterns for adverse event mentions in annotated data. The patterns were then used to find adverse reactions in unlabeled data. However, with manual annotation, the machine learning approach did not result in better performance [15].

After entity recognition, sentences from patient discussions containing both drug and event entities are extracted. Detecting whether the events are associated with the drugs in these sentences is a critical issue in patient social media ADE research. Entity relation extraction, the process of scanning text for relationships between named entities, can help solve this problem. The relation extraction techniques can be categorized into three types: co-occurrence analysis, rule-based approach, and statistical learning approach.

In prior studies, co-occurrence analysis has been predominantly used to extract drug and adverse event relations from user comments because of its simplicity and flexibility [2][14][18][26]. Co-occurrence analysis assumes that if two entities are both mentioned in the same sentence, there is an underlying relationship between them [12]. However, co-occurrence analysis captures little syntactic or semantic information. This approach cannot distinguish true relations when multiple entities appear in one sentence and when negation exists, leading to low precision and accuracy.

More sophisticated relation extraction techniques, such as statistical learning methods, have the potential to increase the precision and accuracy in relation extraction [15]. Statistical learning approaches usually separate relation extraction into two steps: relation detection and relation classification [15]. First, a classification model is trained on the annotated text to learn relation patterns and determine whether two entities in a sentence have a relation. The second classifier is trained to determine the relation type, based on the result of the first classifier. Kernel based statistical learning techniques have shown promise in identifying various social relations such as locations and organizations [1] and gene interactions in the biomedical domain [15]. In particular, Bunescu et al. [1] developed a kernel method with the shortest path between two entities in the dependency graph for relation extraction, which achieved a significant improvement in performance. This method may be suitable for use with the descriptions, which are usually short, found in health-related social media.

2.4   Performance in Prior Patient Social Media Research

Prior studies have taken different approaches to mine drug-related content in patient social media. We analyze their performance and try to identify the best solutions and opportunities for improvement.

Several studies have developed analytical systems for extracting adverse event entities in social media [2][3][13][18]. The best performance values have been achieved by Leaman et al. [13] using a lexicon approach, with results 78.3% in precision, 69.9% in recall and 73.9% in f-measure. A prior study that adopted machine learning approach attained precision of 70.01%, recall of 66.32% and f-measure of 67.96% [18]. Lexicon-based medical entity recognition thus shows the best performance to date. The results in Leaman et al. [13] nonetheless still have the potential to be improved by combining other health lexicons such as the Consumer Health Vocabulary.

2.5   Research Gaps and Questions

Based on our review, we have identified several research gaps. Most prior studies adopted co-occurrence analysis for adverse drug event extraction [2][13][18][26]. However, this approach captures little syntactic or semantic information. As a result, it cannot distinguish true adverse drug events when multiple drugs and events appear in one sentence, leading to significant noise, irrelevant associations, and low precision. The reported ADEs in patient forums can come from diverse sources such as patients' own experiences, stories from other people, news, and research, all of which can result in significant redundancy and noise. However, the adverse drug event extractions in prior studies were based on all the comments related to drugs and adverse events [2][3][13][18][26]. None of them focused on differentiating reports based on patients' own experiences from hearsay. Lexicon-based approaches may also be improved by incorporating and combining additional health lexicons.

In this study, we develop an analytical framework, AZDrugMiner, to extract patient adverse drug event reports from patient forums. We pose the following research questions:

- Can adverse drug event reports based on patient experiences be differentiated from hearsay?
- Can statistical learning based relation extraction techniques identify drug event associations in sentences more accurately than the current co-occurrence based approaches?

3   Research Design

In this section, we describe the proposed AZDrugMiner framework for extracting patient reported adverse drug events in online patient forums, which is illustrated in Figure 1. Major components of this system are detailed in the subsections.

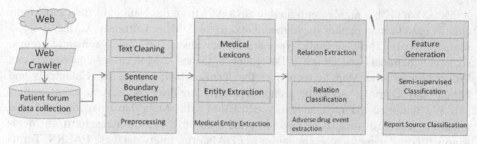

Fig. 1. AZDrugMiner: Framework for Mining Patient-reported ADEs in online Patient Forums

3.1   Patient Forum Data Collection

A critical component of our research design is the need for data. We developed an automated crawler to download web pages from patient forums, and text parsers were written to extract specific fields in the text. We specifically focused on patient profile information and forum discussions. The patient profile information we extract includes a patient profile number (a unique identifier of a registered user), date of birth, diagnosis, signature and gender. The patient discussion information includes post ID (a unique identifier of a post in the forum), URL, topic title, post author's profile number, post data, and post content. Patient profile and discussion data are parsed into specific tables and stored in a data repository for further analysis. Post content is the major focus in this study.

3.2   Preprocessing

After data is collected, it must be processed for further analysis. The preprocessing consists of two steps: text cleaning and sentence boundary detection. Many forum posts contain URLs pointing to external sources and duplicate punctuation. In text cleaning, we formulate rules using regular expressions to remove URLs, duplicate punctuation, and other noise patterns from the forum posts. Forum posts usually are composed of multiple sentences and may cover multiple aspects of a given topic. The sentences may each have different meanings and concepts to convey. In our study, we focus on sentence level information extraction, which takes the sentence as the basic unit from which to extract adverse drug events. We segment a post into sentences using a state-of-the-art open source natural language processing tool, OpenNLP [20].

3.3   Medical Entity Extraction

It is a challenging task to extract medical entities from patient-generated content. Prior studies suggest that a lexicon-based approach is the most appropriate method. We apply multiple types of lexicon sources to extract drug names and adverse events from the text, including UMLS [25], FAERS [9], and CHV [6].

MetaMap [17], a highly configurable Java API from the National Library of Medicine, is used to map patient social media text to the UMLS. Currently, UMLS has 135 semantic types. Those semantic types are further abstracted into 15 semantic groups, such as 'Chemicals and Drugs' , 'Disorders' , 'Genes & Molecular Sequences' , etc. We configure MetaMap to recognize the terms which belong to 'Chemicals and Drugs' and 'Disorder' semantic groups for extracting drug and adverse event entities [2]. We initialize the medical entity extraction with MetaMap to recognize terms matching standard medical lexicons in patient forums. We filter results from Meta-Map with drug names and event names in FDA's drug safety database FAERS. Terms that never appear in FAERS will not be considered in further analysis. Then we extend the entity extraction to include the Consumer Health Vocabulary (CHV) [6], which contains 47,505 UMLS standard medical terms, corresponding to 127,081 consumer-preferred terms. For each term MetaMap identified, we query the CHV to get its consumer-preferred terms and add to our lexicon. The found consumer-preferred terms are used to search for additional entities in the patient forum. All the sentences with both drug and event entities are extracted for further analysis.

3.4 Adverse Drug Event Extraction

When sentences with both drug and event entities are extracted, we need to detect whether the adverse events are associated with the drugs in those sentences. This problem is essentially an entity relation extraction task. Previous studies in patient social media relied on co-occurrence analysis to resolve this, which resulted in low precision and accuracy. Other studies in relation extraction suggested a kernel based machine learning approach to help increase the precision [15]. We propose to apply a kernel based learning method to extract adverse drug events in patient forums. It consists of two steps: relation extraction and relation classification.

Relation Extraction
Relation extraction is an important step in adverse drug event extraction. It aims to detect whether the drug and event in a sentence has a relation. We accomplish relation extraction using shortest dependency path kernel based machine learning method [1], which consists of several components, including: feature generation, kernel function, and classification method.

Feature Generation
Dependency graph provides a representation of grammatical relations between words in a sentence. It has been designed to be easily understood and used to effectively extract textual relations [27]. In the dependency graph, words in the sentence are nodes in the graph and grammatical relations are edge labels. There are 53 different grammatical relations. Among them, the most commonly used are 'nsubj' for nominal subject, 'dobj' for direct object and 'amod' for adjectival modifier [22]. A grammatical relation holds between a governor (also known as a regent or a head) and a

dependent. Figure 2 shows the dependency graph of a sentence. In this sentence, hypoglycemia is an adverse event entity and Lantus is a diabetes treatment. Grammatical relations between words are illustrated in the Figure 2. For instance, 'cause' and 'hypoglycemia' have a relation 'dobj' as 'hypoglycemia' is the direct object of 'cause'. In this relation, 'cause' is the governor and 'hypoglycemia' is the dependent.

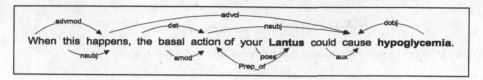

Fig. 2. A sample sentence represented as a dependency graph

Shortest dependency path between two entities is the path from one to the other with minimized words. It offers, in very condensed format, the information needed to assess the relation [4]. A shortest dependency path is represented as a sequence of words with arrows that indicate the orientation of each relation [1]. The shortest dependency path between Lantus and hypoglycemia in the sentence is illustrated in Table 1.

Table 1. Shortest dependency path between a pair of event and drug in sentence

Relation Instance	Shortest Path in Dependency Graph
R(Hypoglycemia, Lantus)	Hypoglycemia -> cause <- action <-Lantus

The shortest dependency path, however, is completely lexicalized and consequently the performance will be limited by data sparsity. We alleviate this by categorizing words into classes with varying degrees of generality and allowing paths to use both words and their classes. Word classes include part-of-speech (POS) tags and generalized POS tags such as Noun and Verb [1][15]. The entity type is also used for the two ends of the shortest path [1]. Shortest path, POS tag, generalized POS tag are extracted using StanfordCoreNLP package [22]. The set of features can be defined as Cartesian product over word classes as illustrated in Figure 3 with the Hypoglycemia and Lantus relation [1].

$$\begin{bmatrix} Hypoglycemia \\ NN \\ Noun \\ Event \end{bmatrix} \times [->] \times \begin{bmatrix} cause \\ VB \\ Verb \end{bmatrix} \times [<-] \times \begin{bmatrix} action \\ NN \\ Noun \end{bmatrix} \times [<-] \times \begin{bmatrix} Lantus \\ NN \\ Noun \\ Treatment \end{bmatrix}$$

Fig. 3. Features generated from dependency graph

The relation instance in Figure 3 can be represented as a sequence of features $X=[x_1,x_2,x_3,x_4,x_5,x_6,x_7]$, where $x_1=\{$Hypoglycemia, NN, Noun, Event$\}$, $x_2=\{->\}$, $x_3=\{$cause, VB, Verb$\}$, $x_4 =\{<-\}$, $x_5=\{$action, NN, Noun$\}$, $x_6=\{<-\}$, $x_7=\{$Lantus, NN, Noun, Treatment$\}$.

Kernel Function

Statistical learning methods such as Support Vector Machines [11] rely on kernel functions to find a hyperplane that separates positive examples from negative. In this study, if $x=x_1x_2...x_m$ and $y=y_1y_2...y_n$ are two relation examples, where x_i denotes the set of features corresponding to position i, the kernel function is computed as in equation below [1][4]:

$$K(x,y) = \begin{cases} 0, m \neq n \\ \prod_{i=1}^{n} c(x_i, y_i), m = n \end{cases} \tag{1}$$

$C(x_i, y_i)=|x_i \cap y_i|$ is the number of common features between x_i and y_i.

Classification

Classification in relation extraction is used to distinguish relation instances with a relation from those without. Transductive Support Vector Machines (TSVM) is a machine learning method that uses hyperplanes to find the maximally distant separation between two classes of data based on the kernel function [11]. SVM-light [23], an open source software package for Transductive Support Vector Machine is adopted in this study because it is widely used in prior studies [14][27] and allows user defined kernels. We modified SVM-light with shortest dependency kernel for SVM-learning.

Relation Classification

Semantic information such as negation or whether the drug is prescribed to treat a disease or causing a disease cannot be captured in shortest dependency path. Thus, relation classification is necessary. The types of relation considered in our research include: negated adverse drug event, true adverse drug event, and drug indication. Table 2 below shows examples for each type.

Table 2. Relation Type Example

Post ID	Content	Relation Type
88270	I haven't [Negation] had any allergic reaction [Event] to Lantus [Drug].	Negated ADE
7724	Well, basically I take Actos 45m, Glucophage, Neurontin [Drug] (pain) [Indication], viagra, and Insulin Shots 30 NPH two times a day and scaled R (10 to 25 units) once a day.	Drug Indication
83068	Now I've read a few posts in this thread that indicate depression [Event] as a possible side effect from Lantus [Drug].	True Adverse Drug Event

We use NegEX [19], an open source Java tool to detect whether an adverse drug event is negated. NegEX focuses on negation identification for clinical conditions based on linguistic rules [6]. It has 531 rules in English for negation identification. Indications of a drug are well-documented in drug safety databases such as FAERS.

Drug indication relations can be identified by comparing the relation instances with indications in the FAERS database where they are well-documented.

3.5 Report Source Classification

Patient social media information can come from different sources. Some are based on patients' own experiences; others emanate from news and stories, which may result in duplication and noise. Classification of the report source is essential because it can filter the ADE reports not grounded on patients' experiences and reduce noise and redundancy. There is no previous patient social media research that addresses this issue. The closest study to our work was a study on classifying authors' product reviews as "personal views" or "impersonal views" [14]. Li et al. [14] used bag of words (BOW) features to classify authors' viewpoints and achieved accuracy of 80%. We borrow the prior study's perspective and develop a machine learning classifier to identify reports based on patient experience. In order to classify the report source of adverse drug events, we develop a feature-based 2-class classification model to distinguish patient reports from hearsay.

Feature Generation

The previous study above used BOW features and resulted in high accuracy [14]. In this study, we extend the BOW features to bigrams and add more syntactic information to test whether we can further improve the performances. Table 3 below shows feature sets for report source classification.

Table 3. Features for report source classification

Feature Sets	Number of Features
Bag of Words	6,254
Bigram	29,898
Bag of Words + POS tag	10,218

Semi-supervised Learning Classification Method

As annotated data is expensive, semi-supervised classification methods such as Transductive SVM, which leverages both labeled and unlabeled data, will be helpful. It can build the model with a small set of annotated data and conduct transductive inference in unlabeled data [11]. In this study, Transductive SVM in SVM-light [23] is used to conduct semi-supervised learning from both labeled and unlabeled data from forum discussions and classify report sources.

3.6 Research Hypotheses

Based on our research design, we propose the following hypotheses:

H1. Statistical learning based adverse drug events association detection in patient forums can be more accurate than co-occurrence analysis based approaches.

H1a. Relation extraction with shortest dependency path kernel will outperform co-occurrence analysis based approaches.
H1b. Adding relation classification to relation extraction model will outperform simple relation extraction model.

H2. Report source classification can accurately identify patient experienced adverse drug events from hearsay.

4   Experiment

4.1   Data

In this study, we investigate the adverse drug events discussion in a well-known diabetes online community (http://community.diabetes.org) which belongs to the American Diabetes Association. A summary of the data is shown in Table 4.

Table 4. Test bed summary

Forum Name	Community.diabetes.org
Number of Posts	185,874
Number of Topics	26,084
Number of Member Profiles	6,544
Time span	2009.2-2012.12
Total Number of Sentences	1,348,364
Average Number of Sentence Per Post	7.25

4.2   Evaluation Metrics

We use standard machine-learning evaluation metrics—accuracy, precision, recall, and f-measure—to evaluate the performance of relation extraction and classification. These metrics have been widely used in information extraction studies [1][15].

4.3   Evaluation

In order to evaluate the performance of our research framework, we manually annotated 200 sentences with both drug and event entities. Table 5 shows the statistics about entities, relations and report source in the annotated data.

Table 5. Statistics about entities, relations and reports source in annotated data

Entity Type	Number of Mentions
Drug	253
Event	224
Relation Type	**Number of Occurrences**
Drug-Adverse Event	124
Drug-indication	21
Negated Drug- Adverse Event	75
No relations	102
Report Source	**Number of Sentences**
Patient Experience	121
Hearsay	79

Medical Entity Extraction

We evaluated the performance of AZDrugMiner on medical entity extraction by comparing the results to manual annotation on 200 randomly selected sentences with at least 2 medical terms. Table 6 shows the performance of Medical Entity Extraction.

Table 6. Evaluation of Medical Entity Extraction

Entity Type	Precision	Recall	F-measure
Drug	93.9%	91.7%	92.5%
Event	87.3%	80.3%	83.5%

The performance of our system surpasses the best performance in prior studies, which is achieved by applying UMLS [24] and MedEffect [16] to extract adverse events from DailyStrength [13]. There may be several causes for this strong performance. Firstly, we combine a standard lexicon with health consumer vocabulary, which increases the recall. Secondly, filtering drug and events that have never appeared in the FAERS drug safety database helps to increase precision. Additionally, DailyStrength [7] is a general health-related social website where users may have a more diverse health vocabulary and more linguistic variety [13].

Based on our evaluation, we can observe that medical entity extraction on event entities attains a lower performance than extraction on drug entities. The major source of error in extracting events is caused by patients' ambiguous descriptions of medical events (e.g., Post_id: 93134, I can sleep through the night without worrying about **a low [Event]** because my Lantus won't adjust for the Dawn Phenomenon.). Medical lexicons generally fail to recognize those entities because they are highly dependent on contextual information in the sentences. This error can be solved by applying semantic analysis in the sentences and building more context-dependent lexicons.

Adverse Drug Event Extraction

To perform adverse event extraction, we manually annotated 200 relation instances. Half contain a relation between drug and event while the other half do not. The remainder of the corpus is unlabeled data. Both labeled and unlabeled data are used to train the Transductive SVM classifier. We evaluate our system by comparing results using co-occurrence analysis (CO) with relation extraction (RE) and relation extraction combined with relation classification (RE+RC). Table 7 below shows the performance of different methods on extracting adverse drug events.

Table 7. Evaluation of Adverse Drug Event Extraction

Method	Precision	Recall	F-measure
CO	38.50%	100%	55.6%
RE	62.1%	56.5%	59.2%
RE+RC	82.0%	56.5%	66.9%

Compared to the co-occurrence analysis approach, relation extraction contributes to an increased precision while leading to low recall. However, overall performance of RE is better than CO. Relation classification can further improve the precision by filtering drug indications and negated ADEs. Based on the evaluation, both H1a and H1b are supported.

Based on the evaluation of adverse drug event extraction, we observe a significant decrease in recall while adopting the kernel-based machine learning method. The low recall is caused by errors in detecting relations in long relation instances. A long sentence has more flexible ways to present a relation. Those long relation representations have low occurrences in labeled data, resulting in a low learning rate and low recall. This issue can be resolved by incorporating active learning [24] , a form of machine learning which determines what relation instances should be labeled for better extraction performance.

Report Source Classification

To perform report source classification, we manually annotated 100 sentences from the training corpus, among which half is from patients' personal experiences and the other half is from hearsay. Both labeled and unlabelled data in the training corpus are used to train a SVM to differentiate personal experience adverse drug event from hearsay. Performance of report source classification is listed in Table 8.

Overall, BOW features achieve the best performance. Bigram and BOW+POS features result in an increase in precision while leading to a decreased recall. BOW features have a more balanced performance. Our model yields a similar accuracy compared to [14]. H2 is supported.

Errors in report source classification mainly happen in long sentences with few pronouns referring to the patients. Errors caused by long sentences may be corrected by using relation extraction to detect the relations between the events and the pronouns in the sentences.

Table 8. Evaluation of Report Source Classification

Feature set	Precision	Recall	F-measure	Accuracy
Bag of Words	83.9%	84.3%	84.1%	80.8%
Bigram	86.4%	77.5%	81.7%	79.0%
Bag of Words+POS	85.2%	79.7%	82.4%	79.6%

4.4   Analysis of ADE Reports in FAERS vs Reports in Patient Forums

We apply the system to the entire forum and compare the extraction results with documented adverse events in FAERS. The adverse event reports from patient forums are from January 2009, when the forum starts to November 2012, our latest data collection. The FAERS reports are from January 2004, when FAERS first started to September 2012.

Similarity between FAERS ADE Reports and Patient Forum ADE Reports
Patient ADE reports extracted by our system share a large number of common ADEs with reports from FAERS. For example, for Byetta, an injectable prescription medication intended to control blood sugar, 6 out of top 10 adverse events in patient reports are consistent with the top adverse events from FAERS. The common ADEs include decrease in weight, nausea, vomiting, diarrhea, pancreatitis, and headache. Other adverse events with smaller proportions in reports are not listed here. Figure 4 below shows the distribution of the common ADEs of Byetta.

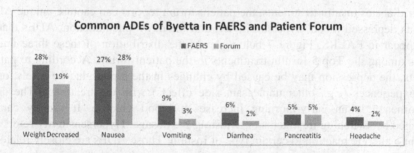

Fig. 4. Common ADEs of Byetta in FAERS and Patient Forum

For drugs with well-known adverse events such as Avandia with Myocardial Infarction, both FDA's reports and social forum reports can highlight Avandia's increased risk for heart disease. Figure 5 below shows the Top 5 common events of Avandia in both patient forums and FAERS.

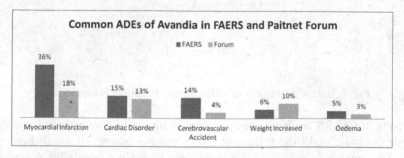

Fig. 5. Common ADEs of Avandia in FAERS and Patient Forum

Difference between FDA's FAERS Reports and Patient Social Forum Reports
For Diabetes oral medications, FDA's reports focus on more serious adverse drug events such as death, renal failure acute etc., while patient social forum reports

contain more mild ADEs, such as weight changes, diarrhea and constipation. Figure 6 shows Top 10 ADEs of Metformin in FAERS and patient forum. Among the Top 10 adverse events from patient forum, five of them consist with top events from FAERS. However, patient reports do not contain severe adverse events such as acute renal failure and metabolic acidosis.

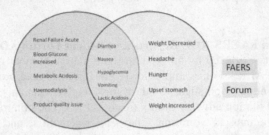

Fig. 6. Contrast of Metformin adverse events from FAERS and Forums

For diabetes insulin treatments, the patient forum reports can capture unique ADEs such as depressed mood, hypersensitivity, and the dawn phenomenon; ADEs that do not appear in FAERS. Figure 7 below shows the distribution of these three unique ADEs among the Top 5 Insulin treatments in the patient forum. According to patient reports, the depression may be caused by changes in the blood glucose levels, or by bad experiences (e.g., other unpleasant side effects) with the treatment. The dawn phenomenon is an early-morning increase of blood glucose. It usually can be managed by switching treatments or adjusting the dosage. Hypersensitivity refers to a patient's allergic reaction to certain type of insulin. Those ADEs are closely related to diabetes treatment management and may reflect patients' needs for more customized regimens.

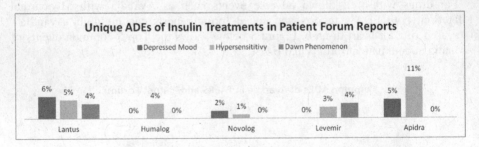

Fig. 7. Unique ADEs of Insulin Treatments in Patient Forum Reports

Reports in FAERS are biased toward drugs with well-known adverse events. For example, Avandia ranks the highest in report number among all the diabetes treatments. The number of reports is still drastically increasing even after Avandia was withdrawn due to the increased risks of heart problem from market beginning in November 2011. However, in the patient forum reports, Avandia ranks only at No.10 in report number, far behind common diabetes treatments such as Metformin and Lantus.

5   Conclusion

In this study, we develop the AZDrugMiner framework to extract patient reported adverse drug events in social media. The proposed statistical learning relation extraction approach improves the performance of adverse drug event extraction. Report source classification filters noisy data and duplication in reports and maintains a set of high quality patient social media adverse drug event reports that are generated based on patient experience.

Based on the information extraction results, we find that patient ADE reports in social media have several advantages: patient social media ADE reports are not biased to severe ADEs; patient reports of ADEs in social media are not biased to drugs with well-known events; and patient ADE reports can capture patients' emotional reactions to treatments. Patient social media ADE reports can help healthcare professionals understand treatment management in a broader context and respond not only to serious ADEs but also to mild events that may affect a larger population.

In this study, we assume that the sentence is the basic unit for adverse drug event association detection. Thus, the relation between an adverse event and a drug across sentences is not considered. We explored the shortest dependency path kernel in relation extraction. However, we did not compare the performance of shortest dependency path kernel with other kernel function such as SubTree kernel and standard tree kernel [27]. Combining multiple kernel functions has the potential to improve the relation detection performance as well [15].We explored the Transductive SVM based semi-supervised machine learning in this study and shown that it can be effective. However, other approaches in conducting semi-supervised learning such as self-training, co-training and others may also be effective. In the future, we will explore other options for a semi-supervised learning framework to further improve the performance.

Acknowledgements. This work was supported in part by DTRA, #HDTRA1-09-1-0058. We also gratefully acknowledge the contribution of Dr. Randall Brown for advices on this study.

References

1. Bunescu, R.C., Mooney, R.J.: A Shortest Path Dependency Kernel for Relation Extraction. In: Proceedings of the Conference on Human Language Technology and Empirical Methods in Natural Language Processing, pp. 724–731 (2005)
2. Benton, A., Ungar, L., Hill, S., Hennessy, S., Mao, J., Chung, A., Holmes, J.H.: Identifying potential adverse effects using the web: A new approach to medical hypothesis generation. Journal of Biomedical Informatics 44(6), 989–996 (2001)
3. Bian, J., Topaloglu, U., Yu, F.: Towards large-scale twitter mining for drug-related adverse events. In: Proceedings of the 2012 International Workshop on Smart Health and Wellbeing, pp. 25–32. ACM (2012)
4. Borgwardt, K.M., Kriegel, H.P.: Shortest-path kernels on graphs. In: Fifth IEEE International Conference on Data Mining, p. 8. IEEE (2005)

5. Chee, B.W., Berlin, R., Schatz, B.: Predicting adverse drug events from personal health messages. In: AMIA Annual Symposium Proceedings, vol. 2011, pp. 217–226 (2011)
6. Consumer Health Vocabulary, http://www.consumerhealthvocab.org/
7. Chapman, W., Hilert, D., Velupillai, S., Kvist, M., et al.: Extending the NegEx Lexicon for Multiple Languages. In: Proceedings of the 14th World Congress on Medical & Health Informatics (2013)
8. DailyStrength, http://www.dailystrength.org/
9. FDA's Adverse Drug Event Reporting System (FAERS), http://www.fda.gov/Drugs/GuidanceComplianceRegulatoryInformation/Surveillance/AdverseDrugEffects/default.htm
10. Jiang, Y.L., Liao, Q.V., Cheng, Q., Berlin, R.B., Schartz, B.R.: Designing and evaluating a clustering system for organizing and integrating patient drug outcomes in personal health messages. In: AMIA Annual Symposium Proceedings 2012, pp. 417–426 (2012)
11. Joachims, T.: Transductive inference for text classification using support vector machines. In: Machine Learning- International Workshop, pp. 200–209 (1999)
12. Kuhn, M., Campillos, M., Letunic, I., Jensen, L.J., Bork, P.: A side effect resource to capture phenotypic effects of drugs. Mol. Syst. Biol. 6, 34 (2010)
13. Leaman, R., Wojtulewicz, L., Sullivan, R., Skariah, A., Yang, J., Gonzalez, G.: Towards Internet- Age Pharmacovigilance: Extracting Adverse Drug Reactions from User Posts to Health-Related Social Networks. In: Proceedings of the 2010 Workshop on Biomedical Natural Language Processing, pp. 117–125. ACL (2010)
14. Li, S., Huang, C.R., Zhou, G., Lee, S.Y.M.: Employing personal/impersonal views in supervised and semi-supervised sentiment classification. In: Proceedings of the 48th Annual Meeting of the Association for Computational Linguistics, pp. 414–423 (2010)
15. Li, J., Zhang, Z., Li, X., Chen, H.: Kernel-based Learning for Biomedical Relation Extraction. Journal of the American Society for Information Sciences and Technology 59(5), 756–769 (2008)
16. MedEffect, http://www.hc-sc.gc.ca/dhp-mps/medeff/index-eng.php
17. MetaMap, http://metamap.nlm.nih.gov/
18. Nikfarjam, A., Gonzalez, G.H.: Pattern mining for extraction of mentions of Adverse Drug Reaction from user comments. In: Proceeding of 2011 AMIA Annual Symposium, pp. 1019–1026 (2011)
19. NegEX, https://code.google.com/p/negex/
20. OpenNLP, http://opennlp.apache.org/
21. PatientsLikeMe, http://www.patientslikeme.com/
22. Stanford CoreNLP, http://www-nlp.stanford.edu/software/dependencies_manual.pdf
23. SVM-Light, http://svmlight.joachims.org/
24. Tong, S., Koller, D.: Support vector machine active learning with applications to text classification. Journal of Machine Learning Research (2000)
25. Unified Medical Language System (UMLS), http://www.nlm.nih.gov/research/umls/
26. Yang, C.C., Yang, H., Jiang, L., Zhang, M.: Social media mining for drug safety signal detection. In: Proceedings of the 2012 International Workshop on Smart Health and Wellbeing, pp. 33–40. ACM (2012)
27. Zelenko, D., Aone, C., Richardella, A.: Kernel methods for relation extraction. Journal of Machine Learning Research 3, 1083–1106 (2003)

Author Index